Young People and Sexual Health

Young People and Sexual Health

Individual, social and policy contexts

Edited by Elizabeth Burtney and Mary Duffy

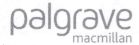

First published 2004 by
PALGRAVE MACMILLAN
Houndmills, Basingstoke, Hampshire RG21 6XS and
175 Fifth Avenue, New York, N.Y. 10010
Companies and representatives throughout the world

PALGRAVE MACMILLAN is the global academic imprint of
the Palgrave Macmillan division of St. Martin's Press, LLC and
of Palgrave Macmillan Ltd. Macmillan® is a registered
trademark in the United States, United Kingdom and other
countries. Palgrave is a registered trademark in the European
Union and other countries.

ISBN 0–333–99357–8

This book is printed on paper suitable for recycling and made
from fully managed and sustained forest sources.

A catalogue record for this book is available from the British
Library.

A catalog record for this book is available from the Library of
Congress.

10 9 8 7 6 5 4 3 2 1
13 12 11 10 09 08 07 06 05 04

Printed and bound in Great Britain by
J. W. Arrowsmith Ltd., Bristol

Contents

v

Figures

Tables

Boxes

Contributors

Susan Batchelor is currently researching her Ph.D. on violent young women detained in prison in Scotland. She has been involved in research since her graduation from the University of Keele in 1997 and her research interests are young offenders, violence and the role of the media. Susan recently completed a groundbreaking piece of research with Jenny Kitzinger that highlighted the messages available in the Scottish media regarding teenage sexuality.

Simon Blake is the Assistant Director of Children's Development at NCB where he leads on Personal, Social, Health Education and Citizenship. Prior to this, he was the Director of the Sex Education Forum. He is a member of the Teenage Pregnancy Strategy Independent Advisory Group, the Sexual Health and HIV Strategy Core Development Group and an assessor for the National Healthy School Standard. Simon has worked with boys and young men in a range of settings and has also trained professionals working with them. He is co-author of *Strides: A Practical Guide to Sex and Relationships Education with Young Men* and *Moving Goalposts: Setting a Training Agenda for Sexual Health Work with Boys and Young Men* – both published by the FPA.

Elizabeth Burtney is a freelance researcher researcher specializing in young people's sexuality. For six years prior to this she was a sexual health research specialist with the Health Education Board for Scotland (HEBS) where she was heavily involved in developing the sexual health strategy on behalf of the Scottish Executive. Her research experience includes evaluation of interventions aimed at improving sexual health in a range of settings including the media, schools and community programmes.

Katie Buston is a senior researcher at the MRC Social and Public Health Sciences Unit at Glasgow University. She has a Ph.D. in Government from Strathclyde University. Katie has worked on the SHARE sex education project since 1996, evaluating a specially designed teacher-led sex education package in 25 Scottish schools. Her research interests include young people, mental health and qualitative methods, as well as sexual health. She has written several articles on gay, lesbian and bisexual youth, as well as on school-based sex education and young people's sexual behaviour.

Judy Corlyon is a senior researcher at the Tavistock Institute working on a variety of projects which include an evaluation of Healthy Living Centres in England, and an evaluation of overseas residential care provided by Save the

Children. She is also joint joint coordinator of the National Teenage Parent Research and Practice Group, and assistant editor of the *Journal of Adolescence*. She has been carrying out research into families and family relationships for many years and most recently has focused on teenage parents and on young people in public care.

Susan Douglas-Scott is the Chief Executive of Phace Scotland, a national HIV and sexual health organization. Prior to this she was the Director of FPA Scotland, previously working in disability services. Her most recent work in disability focuses on sexual health inequalities faced by people with learning difficulties. In 2003 Susan co-wrote two training packs to help staff address sexual health and education with service users. This complements FPA Scotland's wide programme of sexual health training for staff who work with people with learning difficulties.

Mary Duffy is Principal Officer in Barnardo's Policy, Research and Influencing Unit. She manages a portfolio of research in Scotland and northeast England relating to children, young people and their families focusing on health issues. Mary was previously based at the Health Education Board for Scotland and the Health and Safety Executive and she has a D.Phil from the University of Oxford. She has a keen interest in research/practice/policy transfer and evidence-based decision making and has edited a range of publications in this regard.

Simon Forrest is a freelance consultant specializing in young people's sexual health and behaviour. He has previously been Director of the Sex Education Forum and worked in the Department of Sexually Transmitted Diseases, University College London on the RIPPLE study of peer-led sex education in schools. He is also an honorary Senior Lecturer in Adolescent Sexual Health in the Faculty of Health and Social Care Sciences, St George's Hospital Medical School and Visiting Fellow at the Social Science Research Unit based at the Institute of Education within the University of London.

Deirdre Fullerton is a freelance researcher focusing on young people's health including sexual health. Previously she worked for the University of Ulster, University of London and University of York reviewing the evidence base of health and social interventions. Her research interests lie in social inequalities, with a specific focus on teenage pregnancy and sexual health. In 1997 she completed an extensive review of national and international research on the topic of teenage pregnancy which was published in the *Effective Health Care Bulletin*. Her most recent co-authored publication is a practical guide to using the British Social Attitudes data using SPSS entitled *Social Research with SPSS* (Palgrave, 2001).

Marion Henderson is a researcher with the MRC Social and Public Health

Sciences Unit where she works on the SHARE randomized controlled trial to evaluate teacher-delivered sex education. She is currently near completion of a Ph.D. researching school effects on a range of health-related behaviours (alcohol consumption, smoking, drug-use and physical activity). Her research interests include evaluation of health education and health policies, particularly in the fields of sexual health, alcohol and substance-use. She has previously undertaken research for the Medical Research Council (MRC), the World Health Organization, the European Commission, the Scottish Office Education Department, the Economic and Social Research Council and various health boards (community health care NHS trusts).

Alison Hosie is a research associate at Newcastle University where she is involved in a selection of action research projects aimed at pregnancy prevention as well as exploring LEA approaches to re-engaging young mothers and pregnant young women of school age, into education. Alison's qualifications include a B.A. in Social Policy and an M.Sc. in Medical Sociology. Her Ph.D. focused on a comparative policy analysis relating to teenage pregnancy.

Roger Ingham is the Director of the multidisciplinary Centre for Sexual Health Research (www.socstats.soton.ac.uk/cshr), and concentrates on aspects of sexual conduct amongst young people. The centre has carried out research in risk-taking, social and cultural contexts of sexual activity, multi-level modelling of teen conceptions, comparative analyses of sexual conduct in European countries, the relationship between early sexual activity and service use, and worked in developing countries on an advisory basis. Most recently Roger has been involved in the development of the sexual health strategy for England.

Rachel Partridge is a researcher at the Centre for Sexual Health Research, University of Southampton. She is currently leading and coordinating a variety of quantitative and qualitative projects as part of the Safe Passages to Adulthood Programme, a DFID-funded international research programme focusing on young people's sexual and reproductive health in developing countries. An anthropologist by training, she has carried out projects in Africa, Asia and the UK and is now also involved in a research initiative on the research–policy interface.

Hansa Patel-Kanwal OBE is an independent consultant who is currently focusing on organizational development and sexual health work. Prior to this she worked in the voluntary sector as the Director of an HIV and AIDS charity providing culturally and linguistically appropriate services for a range of minority ethnic communities. Hansa is a qualified social worker and has previous experience as a local authority trainer and with policy development in social services. She has co-authored *Let's Talk About Sex and Relationships*, a policy and practice framework for working with children and young people in public care.

She has also produced *Guidelines for Services Providers on Sexual Health Work with Hindu Communities* and compiled *A Positive Woman's Survival Kit,* a resource for HIV positive women living in developing countries.

Martin Raymond is the Head of Public Affairs for NHS Health Scotland (formerly the Health Education Board for Scotland). Formerly a teacher, he has worked in the health field for 15 years and is responsible for the award winning *Think about it* campaign which is aimed at encouraging young people to think about decisions related to their health, including sexual health. He has an MBA from Heriot-Watt University and in 1999 was UK PR Professional of the Year.

Janet Shucksmith is Director of the Centre for Educational Research and Senior Lecturer in Sociology at the University of Aberdeen. Her work centres on issues concerning children's and young people's education, health and social development. She has published extensively on the variations in young people's health behaviours and the relationship of these to family patterns and parenting styles, and her research seeks to enable young people to find a voice in discussing their own health and health education needs. She is currently doing strategic and project-based work relating to child and family wellbeing including educational provision for pre-school children in rural areas, teenage pregnancy and mentoring of vulnerable young people.

Audrey Simpson is the Director of FPA NI and has been for the last 15 years. She has recently completed her Ph.D. in which she looked at the theory and practice of sex education in post primary schools in Northern Ireland. Audrey has written extensively on issues such as sex education, teenage pregnancy and abortion and most recently contributed to two books on women's reproductive rights.

Daniel Wight is a senior researcher for the MRC Social and Public Health Sciences Unit and currently leads an interdisciplinary team which developed a theoretically based teacher-delivered sex education programme (SHARE), in collaboration with the Health Education Board for Scotland. Since 1997 Daniel has been involved in sexual behaviour research and evaluation in Tanzania, in collaboration with the London School of Hygiene and Tropical Medicine. Current interests include young people's lifestyles, parenting, perceptions of risk, HIV/AIDS in developing countries and evaluation.

Ian Young is an international coordinator for the World Health Organization, on secondment from NHS Health Scotland (formerly HEBS) where he championed the Health Promoting School concept in Scotland and was key in producing resources to support this work across Europe. He has been involved in developing teacher capacity to deliver sex education in the classroom and was part of the Scottish Executive review of sex education in Scottish schools linked to the recent repeal of Section 2a in Scotland.

Foreword

Romeo and Juliet: A Parent's Nightmare, A Young Person's Dream?

MARIAN PITTS

This book begins by facing the major dilemma for many of us working with young people in the area of sexual health: are we working with modern day Romeo and Juliet; or should we be ensuring that our young people abstain from the risks and pleasures of sexual behaviour and that we continue to regard romantic attachment as 'puppy love'?

It is strange that, at a time when young people mature earlier and earlier physically, we assert that they are developing much more slowly emotionally and intellectually. The following quotation from a recent discussion of teenage sexuality illustrates this point.

> By the standards of their age, Romeo and Juliet were on the cusp of adulthood.... It's different now, though. Today's 12 and 14 year olds are nowhere near the cusp of adulthood. Most of them have only barely learned to cross the road.
>
> Maureen Freely, *The Times*, 5 September 2003

Despite the fact that we seem to encounter the 'problem' of teenage sex and sexuality on an almost daily basis in our newspapers and other media, there is relatively little well presented work that addresses these issues in an informed and evidence based way. This book does precisely that. Thus it is a timely book – focusing on young people and sexual health from a number of perspectives, and in a variety of ways to ensure that we do not regard 'young people' as an amorphous yet homogenous group.

This book presents quite clearly the evidence that age at first intercourse, and age for first engagement in other sexual activities has consistently declined during the time that we have been measuring it systematically. Currently in Australia we know that some 13 year olds will already be engaged in a variety of sexual activities including genital touching (12.8 per cent) and oral sex (4.8 per cent), while around 25 per cent of 16 year olds will have had sexual intercourse. The figures presented in Chapter 2 indicate clearly that this is also the case in the UK. There we see that the median age at which young people first have sexual intercourse in Britain has fallen from

20 for young men and 21 for young women who were born in the 1930s, to 16 years for both young men and women born in the early 1980s. We need to sit these statistics against those that tell us that the age of marriage has crept steadily upwards, until it is now nearing 30. Thus young people becoming sexually active in today's society can expect around 14 years of sexual experience before they commit 'legally' to a relationship.

So how can we ensure that young people learn to be sexually active in positive and life enhancing ways? At least some of the answers are contained here. The core of the book is an examination of the various layers of influence on the sexual lives of young people. The later parts of the book contain detailed consideration of school-based sex education, of the provision of sexual health services for young people, and of the role of families, peers, culture and media on shaping sexual decision making and lives.

The book also makes visible those young people who have disrupted lives, or who are marginalized from sexual health education through disability or lack of access. It considers the role of religion and of cultures, with particular focus on the Indian, Pakistani and Bangladeshi communities. Most usefully the book emphasizes diversity in teenage sexuality, that there are gay, lesbian and bisexual young people, that for many young people their sexuality is fluid and not necessarily categorical, and that there are many different ways of being a boy – or a girl – in twenty-first century Britain. The book also acknowledges that young people from many cultural and religious backgrounds are part of the United Kingdom.

Analyses of policies concerning sexual health are important since they provide the framework in which our lives are legislated and regulated – and in this book we have perspectives from the United States of America, New Zealand, Australia, the Netherlands, Finland and other European countries. This is a useful context that allows us to view critically the role of national and regional policy within the United Kingdom.

An important element of the book is a human rights perspective, a perspective that is increasingly dominant internationally. The chapter on policy development in the UK introduces us to the perspective of sexual rights and a consideration of the age specific nature of some of these rights. In this context we need a revitalised discussion about the age of consent – more honoured now in its breach; and more generally a discussion of the role of legislation in the area of sexual rights; this book provides some evidence on which to develop this discussion.

I am confident that this book will stimulate debate about sexual health and young people, and that the debate will be better informed from the many useful chapters contained here. Together they bring into profile the urgent need for leadership in the field of sexual health, while not denying the political and cultural sensitivities associated with any changes in this area. But change we must have if we are to help young people to pursue satisfying, safe and happy sexual lives.

Marian Pitts
Professor and Director
Australian Research Centre in Sex, Health and Society
La Trobe University, Melbourne

Part One

Sexuality and Sexual Health in Context

The bigger picture

This book is about the importance of considering the broader context of young people's lives when seeking to understand sexuality and sexual health from their perspective. Policy makers and practitioners increasingly recognize that developing and implementing effective strategies to support young people in making healthy and fulfilling choices and in reducing negative sexual health outcomes requires greater sensitivity to this broader context.

Considering sex and relationships from the point of view of young people means taking account of the factors that influence how they think, act and assign value or priority to issues. It also means accepting that issues may not appear as important to them as they do to adults. Such differing perspectives are particularly relevant when it comes to risk perception.

Risk is a normal part of life. However, it is not an objective concept and the way in which people assess and manage risk varies according to a wide range of psychological, social and cultural factors (Johnson and Covello, 1987; Krimsky and Golding, 1992). Different people view the same situation or action in different ways with respect to the level of risk they attach to it, and some people even actively seek out situations which they recognize as more risky. There are often significant differences between the risk assessments of 'experts' and the lay public, although Golding argues that:

> Public knowledge is no less valuable than expert knowledge and a response that appears rational according to one perspective may be considered quite irrational from the other ... expert knowledge and public knowledge are conditional – each reflects the underlying social relations and implicit assumptions of the various actors.
>
> (Golding, 1992: 24)

The ways in which professionals define and quantify risk may be particularly at odds with the views of young people. And of course parents and teenage children may have conflicting constructions of what constitutes 'risky behaviour'. That said, it is also important to acknowledge the diversity of attitudes and behaviours among young people themselves, and the differing views of risk stemming from the many complex influences on their lives. Young people are not an homogeneous group and the tendency to attribute 'typical' behaviour or to implement blanket strategies to address this behaviour may mean that significant variations are inadequately addressed.

The focus of this section

The chapters in this section describe these wider factors shaping young people's views of sexuality and sexual behaviour, both those impacting within same and opposite sex peer networks and those defining the interactions between young people and adults. They explore issues around the perceived risks attached to certain types of sexual activity and demonstrate how the concept of risk is relevant not just to physical health outcomes but also to reputation, educational attainment, economic prospects and so on. In setting this broader context they provide a foundation upon which subsequent chapters build.

The transition from childhood to adulthood is nowadays more protracted than ever, a kind of extended adolescence characterized for many by increased years in formal education, later entry into employment, and delayed financial independence compared with previous generations. Yet during adolescence many young people still seek to differentiate themselves from the attitudes and behaviours of their parents, striving for independence even while they may still be dependent in many ways. In doing so, they may find themselves in new and challenging situations which offer them a wide range of choices about their behaviours and place upon them different expectations, pressures and constraints regarding appropriate action.

During this transition period in particular, parents may worry about their children's capacity to make safe choices. Fears about smoking, drug-taking, personal safety and the like abound, and general concerns about risk are sometimes amplified by negative media coverage and other social processes (Renn *et al.*, 1992). In relation to sexual health, worries about unintended pregnancy and sexually transmitted infections (STIs) are common, and young women in particular may find themselves under pressure to behave in certain ways. However, despite parental and professional concerns, for many young people the world may seem less threatening, and behaviours that adults might define as excessive or unsafe may seem more like a normal part of life.

Another reason for potential discrepancies in how adults and young people assess situations is that they have different time horizons over which they consider the consequences of actions. For young people, outcomes that are far in the future may be less meaningful, and messages that focus on these long-term outcomes may have limited impact. Thus, while most young people are anxious to avoid pregnancy, the threat from STIs that might cause infertility in one's thirties may seem less real and this in turn may make it more difficult to motivate them to use condoms on top of other contraception.

In considering issues of risk in relation to young people's sexual behaviour, and in thinking about the practice and policy responses required, there is a distinction between 'being at risk' (when some situation or action puts one at risk of a negative outcome) and 'risk taking' (when the people involved are actively choosing to engage in risky activities). It is also important to note how avoidance of risk from the young person's point of view can lead to risk behaviour from a health point of view. For example, fears about the risk to reputation as a result of not knowing how to handle a condom correctly, or worries about being regarded as sexually impotent if not appearing to want sex regardless of context, can lead to unsafe sex.

Issues of reputation and peer appraisal are particularly important within the groups in which young people interact, the same groups through which they learn a lot (not always accurately) about sex. These chapters demonstrate how important such peer groups are in influencing what young people think and how they talk and behave around each other. The fact that much interaction is within same-sex groups (especially prior to first sexual activity with others) is significant, promoting gender-specific understandings of issues relating to sex and relationships, and giving rise to differences between boys' and girls' understandings. Once sexual activity has begun, these gendered perspectives continue to have an important influence, shaping expectations and impacting on young people's views of what is important and appropriate in relation to protecting themselves (or not) with regard to sexual health outcomes.

These chapters remind us that sex is just one aspect of young people's lives, that it is not for them always the most important aspect, and that they do not always view the issues in the same way as those who set pubic health agendas. Their assessment of risk and appraisal of outcomes is shaped by broader aspects of the social and cultural environment, as is their patterns of behaviour with regard to sex and relationships. In trying to support young people to develop healthy sexualities, parents, practitioners and policy makers need to take this into account, above all listening to the voice of young people themselves, since they speak as experts on their own lives.

References

Golding, D. (1992) A social and programmatic history of risk research, in *Social Theories of Risk*, ed S. Krimsky and D. Golding, Westport: Praeger.

Johnson, B. B. and Covello, V. T. (1987) *The Social and Cultural Construction of Risk*, Dordrecht: Reidel.

Krimsky, S. and Golding, D. (eds) (1992) *Social Theories of Risk*, Westport: Praeger.

Renn, O., Burns, W., Kasperson, J. X., Kasperson, R. E. and Slovic, P. (1992) The social amplification of risk: theoretical foundations and empirical applications, *Journal of Social Issues*, **48**(4): 137–60.

1 A Risk Worth the Taking: Sex and Selfhood in Adolescence

JANET SHUCKSMITH

> **Key issues**
>
> - The risks confronting young people in relation to sexual behaviour have changed, but are still real.
> - Risks can seem worth taking when there are pay-offs in terms of developing autonomy, of being able to experiment with identity, of affirming one's transition to adult status.
> - Health education must take heed of these voluntaristic aspects of young people's sexual behaviour.

Overview

This chapter highlights how frequently discussions of young people in relation to sex problematize their behaviour and see it in terms of risks to be avoided and minimized. It describes the importance of understanding the social construction of childhood and transition to adulthood and how these impact on the sexual choices that young people make. It then considers the implications of this for sexual health promotion.

Introduction

Young people reaching sexual maturity these days and deciding whether or not to become sexually active seem – to their parents at least – to be entering a new and risky stage of their lives. Sexual activity has always carried risk: risk of unwanted pregnancy, risk of transmission of infections and, of course, risk to reputation. Thirty years ago we might have assumed that some of these risks were diminishing. Effective and free contraceptive services had been introduced; the social climate had altered. Despite these changes life often looks and feels riskier today than ever. New sexually transmitted infections have arisen or increased in incidence; failures of contraception can seem worse in a society where they interrupt female education and careers; social and sexual reputations still need to be carefully managed, particularly for women. Despite this, young people still feel that this particular transition to adulthood is a risk worth the taking, and, despite the welter of health promotion advice on the topic, often do little to diminish the risk to themselves. Why might this be? How can we seek to understand it?

Perhaps, as Denscombe (2001) advocates, we should be developing an 'alternative perspective', which stops focusing on risk, which does not seek automatically to problematize this aspect of social behaviour, or which does not always construe young people who 'fail' in regard to sexual health as victims. Young people's sexual health is 'framed' in policy in distinct ways. Every policy proposal contains within it an explicit or implicit diagnosis of the 'problem', and the way the problem is represented can shape an issue in ways that limit the possibilities for change (Bacchi, 1999; Tisdall, 2002). The assumption that sexuality is a problem when connected with teenagers begs the question (as Carter (1993) notes in a book review about teenage pregnancy) of whether all is straightforward when we pass the age of 20.

Content analysis of sexual health promotion materials regarding sexual behaviour in young people would undoubtedly reveal the extent to which emphasis has been placed on external influences (peer pressure, family influences, social deprivation, commercial interests, and so on) or personal pathology (low self-esteem, low academic achievement, and so on). Denscombe comments, in relation to his study of young people's smoking behaviour, that 'precious little has been written about the voluntaristic aspects... Rarely has it been asked what benefits young people perceive to be associated [with smoking]' (2001: 159). We could extend this beyond the case of smoking. Precious little work has been published in all health areas that works 'with' rather than 'on' young people, and which makes young people's perspectives a prime focus, as a recent review makes clear (Shucksmith, 2002). Whilst many non-governmental organisations do take the voice of young people on board in developing materials and programmes, these are usually not published in an academic format and give insufficient details of methodology, and so systematic reviews of the literature fail to reflect these insights.

In taking this tack we are not saying that young people do not put themselves at risk, nor that it is wrong for health promoters to do as much as they can to minimize the risks that young people face. What we are saying is that any desire to produce effective health promotion materials or effective interventions must start from where young people are and take account of the ways in which they construct their world. One significant aspect of this is the way in which the concept of risk has become an integral part of the reflexive definition of self for young people in late modernity. We turn now to look at this.

Constructing identity

Many theories of identity formation focus on how people construct an understanding of themselves in relation to others, concentrating on ideas of consistency, continuity, sameness and difference (Jenkins, 1996). Weeks clarifies:

> Identity is about belonging, about what you have in common with some people and what differentiates you from others. At its most basic it gives you a sense of personal location, the stable core to your individuality. But it is also about your social relationships, your complex involvement with others.
>
> (Weeks, 1991: 88)

For all of us, critical parts of our self-identity stem from structural factors like our gender, our class, our race, our nation and so on. In the past, small, homogeneous and slowly changing societies provided a firm (if narrow) foundation for building meaningful identity. In fact identities were almost 'given' and people took what felt like their 'natural place' in the order of things. This sounds like a good description of an Amish community, and a very poor description of the late modern world in which today's teenagers grow up. Today the old certainties about class have withered with the manufacturing and extractive industries that spawned them. Definitional notions of gender have fractured, and large scale patterns of international migration and resettlement create crises of ethnic identity for the Birmingham-born sons and daughters of Caribbean mothers, or the British Muslim children of refugees from the Indian sub-continent. The period we live in has become one of enormous self-reflection upon identity.

Modern societies are diverse, fast-moving and complex and 'offer only shifting sands on which to build a personal identity' (Macionis and Plummer, 2002: 168). Flexibility and the ability to adapt to changing circumstances, the willingness to shift – these all become markers of worth rather than the grounds for suspicion that they would have been in traditional societies. Riesman (1970) would describe people with such aptitudes or inclinations as 'other-directed' rather than 'tradition-directed'. They are willing to try on new identities, new 'selves', almost like people trying on clothing. They will perform in different roles depending on the setting in which they find themselves (Goffman, 1959). Identity in other words is fractured or fragmented. We all search for new frameworks of self-understanding. Giddens talks about all this as a reflexive self-identity:

> Because of the 'openness' of social life today, the pluralization of contexts of action and the diversity of 'authorities', lifestyle choice is increasingly important in the construction of identity and daily activity. Reflexively organised life planning ... becomes a central feature of the structuring of self-identity.
>
> (Giddens, 1991: 5)

As Miles *et al.* (1998) note, young people are 'more adept at, and more willing than adults, to experiment with their identities, no matter what boundaries (whether they be of class, gender or race) of identity may appear to constrain them' (Miles *et al.*, 1998: 83). Part of this trying on of identities by young people is clearly visible in styles of dress and makeup, but is also evidenced in patterns of consumption, and in lifestyle choices around health issues (Pavis *et al.*, 1998). What meaning does sexual activity then hold for young people? Is it possible that sexual behaviour is also used in this shaping of identity?

This does not mean, as Denscombe (2001) points out, that structural factors like class, gender and race play no part or have no influence, but that agency and choice become far more influential than hitherto. Not all authors are happy with this diminution of attention to the structural factors that shape young people's lives (Furlong and Cartmel, 1997). Talking about young people as 'agentic', and discussing their freedom to try on lifestyles can imply that all young people have equal freedom to experiment and 'play' with identity. Those who work closely with young people from minority ethnic groups or with those who live in poverty are quick to point out that this does not apply evenly across the board. Empirical evidence emerging from the many studies funded by the Joseph Rowntree Foundation in the last five years demonstrates the grip that poverty still has on children's and young people's lives. We need to be clear that young people are not a homogeneous group. Ann Phoenix's study of teenage mothers (1991) makes this very clear. Her dismissal of the simplistic notion that those who become pregnant at a very young age are necessarily ignorant, powerless or despairing is coupled with her willingness to listen to young women's own voices. She shows that, for many young women living in poverty, early motherhood is not perceived as damaging their chances. For some, it is an opportunity to make the transition out of the rather desperate circumstances of the parental home and make a new start. Most young girls in her study had such poor anticipated opportunities already in educational or career terms that the addition of a small child did not significantly disadvantage them, and occasionally acted as a spur to re-engage them with education.

A difficult boundary

The difficulty involved in young people being allowed to make choices for themselves is perhaps more problematic in relation to sexual behaviour and sexual health than to any other area of their health-related behaviours. In this domain the difficult boundary between child and adult seems more confused than ever. In the same way as young drinkers see themselves making a transition into 'drinking societies' and feel that they must prepare themselves in appropriate ways (Kloep *et al.*, 2001), so many young people see themselves moving towards an adult world which is highly sexualized. Many aspects of this reach down to even our youngest children, with the clothing and music industries, for example, deliberately inducting young people into sexualized thinking and patterns of activity via provocative clothing and boy bands deliberately packaged for the pre-teen female.

Marina Warner in her 1994 Reith lectures commented:

The portraits of the French or English aristocracy and gentry showing children clothed as adults, with jewels and powdered wigs and crinolines and farthingales, were displaying the status of their families; but the little girl in a black dress, patent pumps, lipstick and earrings who was brought out in the finale of a recent Chanel collection was showing off her body, and looked like a travesty of the sex-free youth children are supposed to enjoy.

(Warner, 1994: 46)

Over the past century, there has been, as Morrow and Richards (1996) point out, a trend towards earlier puberty, with age at first menarche declining from between 16 and 17 in the mid-nineteenth century to just under 13 in 1960. Since then there is little evidence of further change. The onset of puberty will thus occur while some girls are still at primary school. At the same time, changes in fashion also now dictate that young women strive for the slim, or even waif-like appearance of the 12 year old, and the mature fashion and pop icons sporting these size 6 figures are often highly sexualized in their presentation, their celebrity antics now the meat and drink of teenage comics, magazines and television reports. It is little wonder then that the boundaries between childhood and adulthood seem to be so difficult to discern and then to negotiate.

Many parents are happy to allow their pre or barely pubescent daughters to copy these pop divas into the realms of sporting provocative underwear, the copying of highly provocative dance routines and so on. Young people may not be able to recognize or handle the reactions that this behaviour can provoke in others – their physical maturity runs well ahead of their emotional maturity.

Despite our general tolerance at societal level for such precocious induction into a sexualized world, we occasionally break out into the most prurient expressions of alarm when young people are taught directly about sex at school. This limits the ways in which young people can be taught about sex, so for instance, discussion about 'safer sex' may be sanitized and limited to discussion of condom use. As Hillier *et al.* (1998) point out, this leaves unnamed other ways of being sexual which are potentially available to young people. Exclusive focus on condoms as protections from sexually transmitted infections (STIs) and pregnancy also 'overlooks the more proximal risk of a sullied reputation, which may be exacerbated through the process of obtaining condoms and, by association, planning for sex' (Hillier *et al.*, 1998: 16). So, to caricature this position somewhat by using a military metaphor, we are prepared at a societal level to place our children in the firing line vis-à-vis their sexuality, but not prepared to give them the armour they need to protect themselves when the bullets start flying.

No-one captures this ambivalence better than Foucault (1984), for whom the history of sexuality in the west since the seventeenth century is a long process of 'turning sex into discourse'. As Cox (1996) notes, one of the most important of these emerging discourses was concerned with the sexuality of children and young people. Discourses for Foucault are strategies for the exercise of power. They define what can be said and what we must be silent about. Central to discourses about young people's sexuality is a denial of that sexuality, but one of the possible consequences of that denial is that childhood and youth are eroticized (Cox, 1996: 135).

Young people seem caught in the middle of our own ambivalence about what childhood is. As Warner says:

> Many of these problems result from the concept that childhood and adult life are separate when they are in effect inextricably intertwined. Children aren't separate from adults, and unlike Mowgli or Peter Pan, can't be kept separate; they can't live innocent lives on behalf of adults, like medieval hermits maintained at court by libertine kings to pray for them, or the best china kept in tissue in the cupboard.
>
> (Warner, 1994: 48)

Making choices, being autonomous, being risky

Part of the transition across the boundary from child to adult is clearly concerned with the development of autonomous action. The expression of choice through consumption is often felt by young people as a form of autonomy (Shucksmith, 2002), and risk-taking is often associated with autonomy. Denscombe highlights this well in the discussion of his empirical data from young people about their risk-taking through smoking:

> Smoking says something about themselves to themselves. It says things like 'I'm in control of my own life' and 'I'm special'. And it is this latter role for smoking which is perhaps a reflection of the self-determination image that ties in with the contemporary social ethos.
>
> (Denscombe, 2001: 174)

But this exercise of autonomy is an essentially risky business. Choice can seem like a fine thing. As adults we would be severely displeased if, setting out to buy a house, for instance, we thought that our choice would be constrained by someone else's view of what was suitable for us. We might soon realize, however – unless someone is kind enough to give us some strong hints – we might well make the 'wrong' choice, wasting our money and our time and saddling ourselves with a property which is quaint but uninsurable, or grand and spacious, but too expensive to heat.

In the realm of sexual autonomy and choice, freedom from past constraints about pregnancy or social disapproval can make modern life seem kinder, but, it could be argued, the lack of constraints and rules exposes us to a higher probability of making 'expensive mistakes'.

Moreover, sexual autonomy is a condition which few young women achieve, since, despite the fact that they are expected to behave with greater emotional maturity, there are still expectations that women will be sexually naive. On the basis of a study exploring the way in which adolescents are represented in the text of health advice and information material, Aapola (1997) concludes:

> This comes up in the school textbooks as well as in the advice manuals. Girls are to behave in 'responsible' way: take good care of themselves and others ... act rationally in sexual contacts, among other things. Rights, experiments and manifestations of autonomy and freedom usually linked with increasing age seem more ambiguous for girls. Dominant discourses of female adolescence emphasize vulnerability and responsibility, which corresponds with traditional discourses of femininity. Male adolescence is linked more with uncontrollability and irresponsibility.
>
> (Aapola, 1997: 64)

The young women in Hillier *et al.*'s study confirm the difficulties they face in negotiating condom use with their partners and in maintaining sexual reputation in a rural environment. Faced with these difficulties their discussions reveal a range of alternative strategies, not least of which is convincing themselves that they are invulnerable, and also trusting in reputation, appearance or the quality of the relationship as a protection against disease. Safe sex methods based on informal sexual history taking (facilitated through gossip) were regarded therefore as providing reliable protection from STIs.

Mitchell and Wellings (1998) raise similar problems about power and autonomy in relationships in discussing young people's accounts of first sexual relationships. Much of the early qualitative work on this comes from a decade ago (Holland *et al.*, 1990, Wight, 1992). These early studies exposed the fact that communication is difficult for young couples, and that the discourse of safer sex is at odds with cultural ideologies of romance and spontaneity. Mitchell and Wellings' more recent investigation with 29 young people at four different locations in England confirms this theme. In their study young people spoke of many of the first sexual encounters taking place in silence, especially when first intercourse took place at a young age. The speed and silence of these events precludes negotiation about safer sexual practices or contraceptive use. The authors found the young men in the sample were more prepared for first intercourse and more likely to carry condoms, and use this finding to suggest that it may be time for education campaigns to refocus towards young men rather than young women.

Conclusion

This short chapter has attempted to explore some elements of the broader context within which young people's lives now unfold, as a background to the chapters that follow, which focus more specifically on issues of sexual behaviour.

Young people's sexuality and sexual behaviour is invariably constructed as a 'problem' in policy and in health promotion discourse. Unwanted or unplanned sexual activity can undoubtedly have unhappy consequences. However, it may be unhelpful in terms of the design of health promotion interventions to ignore the fact that, for many young people, sexual activity is not a problem in itself, but is more likely to be used as a way of finding an answer to problems about identity. As Denscombe (2001) points out, we need to look at the issue from the voluntaristic point of view; what do young people get out of the activity. Why is the risk worth taking?

In trying to answer this question we have looked at how many health behaviours are now part of the construction of identity in an age where there are fewer fixed roles and trajectories for young people. Experimentation is the norm.

It has become unfashionable to talk about youth transition, since it implies that children and young people are in some way 'unfinished' and incomplete, 'becomings' rather than 'beings' (James *et al.*, 1998). Nonetheless the boundaries between childhood, adolescence and adulthood are particularly difficult territory where matters of sexual conduct are concerned. The Rousseau-ian notion of childhood as some sort of 'protected space – a magic garden' is continually under threat from forces which thrust images of a highly sexualized nature into children's lives. Being sexual is so clearly identified with adult status and autonomy that it is almost inevitable that it becomes one of the rites of passage to adulthood.

Becoming autonomous – in this sphere as in others – is not straightforward or without risk. For some the risks are greater than for others, and girls and young women, in particular, still play a more dangerous game than their male counterparts when they gamble with their health or their reputation by sexual risk-taking. Most young people, however, emerge from this period of their lives no worse for wear, despite the anxieties they cause their parents and carers on the way! There is not space in this short chapter to explore the exotic combinations of lust, love and curiosity that compel young people to decide that it is a risk worth the taking. However, it would certainly repay the effort of the determined health promoter to balance the rationality of theories of health change with a more intensive and grounded consultation with young people themselves that allows them to reflect dimensions of their lived experience of intimacy and identity formation.

References

Aapola, S. (1997) Mature girls and adolescent boys? Deconstructing discourses of adolescence and gender. *Young* 5(4): 50–68.
Bacchi, C. (1999) *Women Policy and Politics: The Construction of Policy Problems*. London: Sage.
Carter, P. (1993) Book review in *Youth and Policy* 40: 89–92.

Cox, R. (1996) *Shaping Childhood: Themes of Uncertainty in the History of Adult–Child Relationships*. London: Routledge.

Denscombe, M. (2001) Uncertain identities and health-risking behaviour: the case of young people and smoking in late modernity. *British Journal of Sociology* **52**(1): 157–77.

Foucault, M. (1984) *The History of Sexuality, Volume 1: An Introduction*, trans. R. Hurley. Harmondsworth: Penguin.

Furlong, A. and Cartmel, F. (1997) *Young People and Social Change: Individualisation in Late Modernity*. Buckinghamshire: Open University Press.

Giddens, A. (1991) *Self Identity and Late Modernity*. Cambridge: Polity Press.

Goffman, E. (1959) *The Presentation of Self in Everyday Life*. Garden City, NY: Anchor Books.

Hillier, L., Harrison, L. and Warr, D. (1998) 'When you carry condoms all the boys think you want it': negotiating competing discourses about safe sex. *Journal of Adolescence* **21**: 15–29.

Holland, J., Ramazanoglu, C., Scott, S., Sharpe, S. and Thomson, R. (1990) 'Don't die of ignorance? I nearly died of embarrassment.' Condoms in context, *WRAP Working Paper 2*. Tufnell Press.

James, A., Jenks, C. and Prout, A. (1998) *Theorising Childhood*. Oxford: Polity Press.

Jenkins, R. (1996) *Social Identity*. London: Routledge.

Kloep, M. Hendry, L. B., Ingesbrigtsen, J. E., Glendinning, A. and Espnes, G. A. (2001) Young people in "drinking" societies? Norwegian, Scottish and Swedish adolescents' perceptions of alcohol use. *Health Education Research* **16**(3): 279–91.

Macionis, J. J. and Plummer, K. (2002) *Sociology: A Global Introduction*. 2nd edition. Harlow: Pearson Education.

Miles, S., Cliff, D. and Burr, V. (1998) Fitting in and sticking out: consumption, consumer meanings and the construction of young people's identities. *Journal of Youth Studies* **1**(1): 81–96.

Mitchell, K. and Wellings, K. (1998) First sexual intercourse: anticipation and communication. Interviews with young people in England. *Journal of Adolescence* **21**(6): 717–26.

Morrow, V. and Richards, M. (1996) *Transitions to Adulthood: A Family Matter?* York: Joseph Rowntree Foundation.

Pavis, S., Cunningham-Burley, S. and Amos, A. (1998) Health-related behavioural change in context: young people in transition. *Social Science and Medicine* **47**(10): 1407–18.

Phoenix, A. (1991) *Young Mothers*. Cambridge: Polity Press.

Riesman, D. (1970, originally 1950) *The Lonely Crowd: A Study of the Changing American Character*. New Haven, CT: Yale University Press.

Shucksmith, J. (2002) Young people and health in Scotland: what matters to young people about their health and well-being? *Research in Brief Series no. 3*. Health Education Board for Scotland, Edinburgh.

Tisdall, K. (2002) Constructing the problem, constructing the solutions: young people's health and wellbeing in Scottish Executive policies. *Research in Brief Series*. Health Education Board for Scotland, Edinburgh.

Warner, M. (1994) *Six Myths of Our Time; Managing Monsters*. Reith Lectures. London: Vantage.

Weeks, J. (1991) *Against Nature: Essays on History, Sexuality and Identity.* London: Rivers Oram Press.

Wight, D. (1992) Impediments to safer heterosexual sex: a review of research with young people. *AIDS Care* **4**: 11–12.

Wight, D. (1994) Boys' thoughts and talk about sex in a working class locality of Glasgow. *Sociological Review* **42**: 703–37.

2 The Diversity of Young People's Heterosexual Behaviour

DANIEL WIGHT and MARION HENDERSON

Key issues

- At a given age the extent of young people's heterosexual experiences, and the meanings that they have, vary considerably: national averages obscure this diversity.
- Young people's sexual behaviour is shaped by childhood experiences, current social circumstances and their expectations of the future, but their condom use is primarily shaped through their interaction with their sexual partners.
- Initial heterosexual experiences are entered into with an understanding that is highly gender-specific, largely shaped through same-sex peer groups. This perspective is modified as individuals gain experience of the opposite sex.

Overview

This chapter describes the diversity of young people's heterosexual experiences and explores the main social influences underlying these behaviours. One of the most important dimensions of sexual diversity – sexual orientation – is addressed specifically elsewhere in this book.

Introduction

Young people's sexual behaviour exemplifies Britain's pluralistic society, varying considerably by social class, educational level, ethnicity and religion. In exploring this heterogeneity, the chapter draws mainly on two quantitative and two qualitative studies:

- The National Survey of Sexual Attitudes and Lifestyles (NATSAL) used face-to-face and self-complete questionnaires in 1990–1 with 16–59 year olds (N=18,876) (Johnson *et al.*, 1994; Wellings *et al.*, 1994; Wellings

15

and Mitchell, 1998). It was repeated between 1999 and 2001, using computer assisted questionnaires, with 16–44 year olds (N=11,161) (Wellings *et al.*, 2001).

- SHARE is a longitudinal survey following teenagers in the east of Scotland from age 13/14 to 20, in order to evaluate a specially designed sex education programme (Wight *et al.,* 2002). The chapter uses data from self-complete questionnaires administered in 25 schools, first in 1996 and 1997 (mean age 14 years, 2 months, N=7,616) and then two years later (mean age 16 years, 1 month, N=5,854).
- The Women, Risk and AIDS Project (WRAP) conducted in-depth interviews with 148 16–21 year old women in Manchester and London, between 1988 and 1990 (Holland *et al.*, 1998). The same team conducted a similar Men, Risk and AIDS Project, with 46 men in London being interviewed.
- A study in a working class locality of Glasgow in the early 1990s involved in-depth interviews, group discussions and ethnographic research with 14–16 year old boys (Wight, 1994), and in-depth interviews with 58 19 year old men (Wight, 1996).

Young people's heterosexual behaviour

Start of heterosexual activity

Many young people start engaging in activities such as kissing using tongues from the age of 13 or 14 (Johnson *et al.*, 1994; Henderson *et al.*, 2002). There generally follows a progression of sexual activities leading to vaginal intercourse (Figure 2.1). Oral sex does not appear to be part of the progression of sexual activities: about a quarter of those who reported having had sexual intercourse did not report oral sex. The special nature of oral sex probably reflects the lack of physical intimacy within many young people's sexual relationships, even when they engage in vaginal intercourse, the deeply held association of the genitals (particularly the vagina) with dirt, and young women's inabilities to express their physical desires (Holland *et al.*, 1998). These barriers to oral sex restrict its potential as a 'safer sex' alternative to vaginal intercourse.

The timing, and number of partners involved, in gaining sexual experiences vary considerably. Figure 2.1 presents the levels of sexual experience for two contrasting groups in the SHARE sample: those with the highest likelihood of sexual experience and those with the lowest defined by the main social factors independently associated with early sexual activity. At the age of 16, most of the high likelihood group have engaged in 'heavy petting' (defined as 'hand touching genitals/private parts'), oral sex and vaginal intercourse, while amongst the low likelihood group only half have experienced heavy petting and less than a quarter sexual intercourse. At age 14 more boys than girls reported experiencing different sexual activities

(Henderson *et al.*, 2002) but this had reversed by the age of 16, as found in Norway (Jakobsen, 1997).

Age at first intercourse

The median age at which young people first have sexual intercourse in Britain has fallen from 21 for women and 20 for men born in the early 1930s (Johnson et *al.*, 1994) to 16 for both sexes born in the early 1980s (Wellings et *al.*, 2001). Most of this dramatic change came in the 1950s, and is probably due to a combination of socio-cultural influences, such as changes in women's employment, legislation about sex and improved access to contraception, particularly the pill, as well as the biological factor of reduced age of menarche.

These summary findings tend to disguise the heterogeneity of young people's sexual experiences. For instance, although half of the 16–19 year olds in the second NATSAL reported that they had first had sexual intercourse at or below the age of 16, a tenth reported having had sex at 14 or younger and a tenth at 19 or not at all (Wellings *et al.*, 2001). Ten years earlier a quarter had not had sex by the age of 19 (Johnson *et al.*, 1994).

The younger intercourse is experienced, the more likely it is to have features generally regarded as negative. In NATSAL these were lack of contraception, regret that it happened too early, greater peer pressure and more evidence of

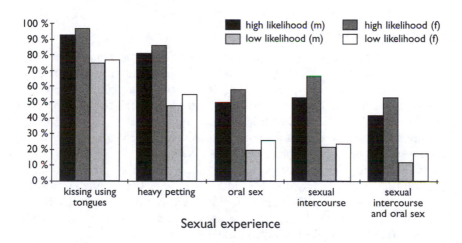

Figure 2.1 Reported sexual experiences at mean age 16 years, 1 month, by groups with 'high' and 'low' likelihood of sexual experience

Note: High likelihood: those who are in at least two of the following groups: highest third spending money, lowest third parental monitoring, not living with both biological parents. Low likelihood: those who are in the lowest third for spending money, highest third for parental monitoring and who are living with both biological parents.
Source: own analysis of SHARE data

coercion by the male partner (Wellings *et al.*, 2001), while in SHARE they were lack of contraception (see Appendix 1 for more detail), regret that it happened too early, greater relative age of sexual partner and shorter duration of the relationship prior to sex.

Amount of sexual activity

The public health and media focus on age of first intercourse and number of sexual partners often obscures the low frequency of sexual intercourse amongst teenagers, both in absolute terms and in relation to adults. Few data on number of sexual partners by specific ages have been published, since findings are usually presented by age bands. Nevertheless, surveys suggest that more than half of 18 year olds have had only one or two sexual partners (Johnson *et al.*, 1994; West *et al.*, 1993), and the amount of sexual activity within these relationships tends to be low (Wight, 1996).

This picture of limited sexual experience is confirmed even amongst the minority of young people who have sex before the age of 16. In the SHARE study, of the 37 per cent of 16 year olds who reported having had sexual intercourse (31 per cent boys, 41 per cent girls), 34 per cent had done so less than three times in the last year and 58 per cent less than ten times. Twenty percent had only had sexual intercourse once and 33 per cent reported only one partner. However, 22 per cent of boys and 17 per cent of girls had had more than five partners.

Contraceptive practice

Young people's use of contraception is more widespread than in any other age group, older people being more likely to want children, to be pregnant or to be sterile (Johnson *et al.*, 1994). However, young people's contraceptive use is partial and less likely, the younger they are when they first have sex (Wellings *et al.*, 2001; West *et al.*, 1993).

There is a clear historical trend towards increased contraceptive use amongst the young (Johnson *et al.*, 1994; Wellings *et al.*, 2001), so that in the SHARE study even amongst 14 year olds less than 20 per cent took no precautions at first intercourse (Henderson *et al.*, 2002). Furthermore, in contrast to past surveys (West *et al.*, 1993), men are now no more likely than women to report not using any contraception; in fact if anything the gender pattern has reversed (Wellings *et al.*, 2001).

Table 2.1 shows that the most common form of protection used by teenagers is the condom (Johnson *et al.*, 1994; West *et al.*, 1993). Few girls use the contraceptive pill before the age of 16, both because it involves anticipating sexual intercourse, when at this age it is generally infrequent and spasmodic, and because it requires medical consultation.

Once young people are in what they regard as a long-term relationship (which can be after a few days or a few months), they tend to move from

Table 2.1 Precautions taken at first and most recent sexual intercourse, reported at mean age 16 years, 1 month (%)

	First intercourse		Most recent intercourse	
	Male	Female	Male	Female
None	14	14	13	15
Withdrawal	7	7	9	8
Condom just before ejaculation	1	2	2	3
Condom throughout	70	68	65	54
Pill	15	13	21	32
Condom and pill	10	9	10	13
Emergency contraception	4	7	3	4
N	732	1096	617	997

Source: own analysis of SHARE data

condom use to the pill (Holland et al., 1998). This is because unwanted pregnancy is still perceived, correctly, to be far more likely than HIV infection, and knowledge of other, far more prevalent sexually transmitted diseases (such as chlamydia) is very poor.

Gender related influences on young people's sexuality

Gender

Sexuality is not a purely innate impulse of which we gradually become aware. Rather it is, to a large extent, learnt, and learnt differently according to gender, for biological and social reasons. Young men's first sexual experiences are usually on their own, masturbating, while young women's are usually with a partner. This is probably connected with boys' much greater familiarity with their genitals, because they are physically far more obvious and because boys regularly handle their penises to urinate. These different initial sexual experiences probably contribute to young men's sexuality being highly embodied, with a focus on genital pleasure and orgasm, while for young women the meaning of sex is bound up more with relationships.

However, the profound gender differences in sexual understanding are largely attributable to the way most young people grow up in sexually segregated social worlds, especially in the period prior to early sexual relationships. In Britain young people see friends as one of the most important sources of information on sex (Johnson et al., 1994; Todd et al., 1999), only recently falling into second place behind schools (Wellings et al., 2001).

Since social activities in the early teens are usually highly segregated by gender (Wight, 1994), the meanings given to sex and sexual relationships come from same-sex peers, thus allowing for a considerable gulf to develop between boys' and girls' understandings. For young men there is the concept that males are sexual creatures and that an interest in sex is understandable, even expected. For young women sex is problematic: it involves serious risks and too much overt interest in sex, particularly if not within established relationships, continues to be seen as not properly feminine.

This is exacerbated by the way young people's self-valuation is shaped much more by the opinions of their own sex than by those of the opposite sex (Gagnon and Simon, 1974), and contact with the opposite sex is perhaps most valued as a key way of developing one's own gender identity (Wight, 1994).

> DW: 'Is it just personality rather than looks [that's important]?'
> R1: 'I don't know, both. You're looking for looks in a bird if you want to show her off, I suppose.'
> DW: 'So who would you show her off to?'
> R1: 'All your pals, take her up the town and that.'
> DW: 'But if you took her up the town your pals are not likely to see her are they?'
> R1: 'Aye, I know, but other boys, they're like that: "Look at her!"'
> R2: 'Look at that wee dick beside her, too!'
>   [Group discussion, 16 year old Glaswegian boys]

Furthermore, one's sexual identity generally develops well after one's gender identity and roles have been established, and the latter shapes the former. To simplify crudely, where conventional gender roles are the norm, young women experience sexual activity as an element of their caring role, while young men experience it as a form of achievement (Gagnon and Simon, 1974).

The intimacy that people seek in heterosexual relationships means that exclusively masculine or feminine perspectives of sexuality are gradually broken down with age. However, the extent to which this happens varies, largely shaped by the predominant gender roles within particular sections of society. For instance, in the Men, Risk and AIDS Project some young men suggested that their fathers still primarily identified with the male peer group at work (Holland *et al.*, 1998). Nevertheless, 'the development of an intimate relationship with a woman is a means by which many of them are able to distance themselves from the values of their male peers irrespective of class, ethnicity or other differences' (Holland *et al.*, 1998: 90).

Gendered power and discourses

Young people seek various things from sexual relationships: intimacy, excitement, higher social status, sexual pleasure, economic security, and so on. Differences in the importance attached to these goals, and in the degree to which young people feel they can openly admit to these goals, can cause power imbalances in relationships, enabling one partner to take and maintain more control over a range of decisions (Tschann *et al.*, 2002). These imbalances may be bolstered by social norms about gender roles and the meaning of sexual relationships.

The way young people talk about their sexual relationships, in what analysts refer to as 'discourses' (Hollway, 1984), can also reflect and nurture power imbalances. Several such discourses of sexuality have been identified (Hollway, 1984; Wight, 1996; Holland *et al.*, 1998), the most important being the 'predatory discourse', used primarily by young men, and the 'romantic discourse', used primarily by young women.

Predatory discourse

The predatory discourse reproduces the stereotype of masculine sexuality and remains prevalent amongst younger men in male-dominated social worlds. Sex is valued primarily as a way of establishing one's masculine identity with one's male peers by having as many sexual partners as possible; physical sexual pleasure is of less importance. The discourse puts teenage boys under considerable pressure to lose their virginity (Wight, 1994) and leads to sex being viewed as a hunt. The less accessible a woman is, the greater one's esteem in seducing her:

> I like a challenge, I'd rather go with somebody they'd say: 'You've got no chance with her', rather than go with some daft slut that anybody could go with – I've never done that. Anybody like that I've always said 'No way, I'd rather go without', know what I mean? I'd rather have a bit of a challenge.
>
> [19 year old man]

There is little value in continuing a sexual relationship once one has 'had it', and so the predatory discourse gives rise to short-term relationships with minimal commitments intended by the man.

Although the predatory discourse is typically used by young men, some young women also adopt it, legitimated by feminist challenges to the sexual double standard. However, despite such challenges and social change more generally, those young women who use this discourse, which strays from the accepted norm, still risk being denigrated as deviant.

Romantic discourse

The romantic discourse incorporates the central ideas and practices of monogamy and partnership and is the predominant way in which young women discuss sexual relationships (Sharpe, 1985; Griffin, 1985; Holland *et al.*, 1998; McRobbie, 2000). In this discourse, sex is understood as a symbol of intimacy with, and commitment to, one's partner, and a couple's first sexual intercourse is primarily valued as a confirmation of how intimate they have become (Kent *et al.*, 1990). Sex is seen to result from being 'swept away' in the romance of the situation, rather than from physical desire. Holland *et al.* (1998: 100) quote a young woman:

> Sex to me is special. It is something that two people who are crazy about each other do, not two strangers that happen to be blind drunk.

Attracting and keeping a boyfriend are central concerns in this discourse, in which boyfriends 'represent social success and status, a secure symbol of acceptable femininity, someone with whom to share experiences and tentatively explore love and sexuality, someone to take them out and give them a good time' (Sharpe, 1985: 214).

The romantic discourse requires women to do the emotional work of maintaining the relationship, while young men often speak of limiting their commitments (Wight, 1996). This can leave young women emotionally vulnerable, and more anxious than men about the impact of not acquiescing to their partner's preferences. For example, while the SHARE study found a broadly similar pattern of sexual experience between the sexes at age 15/16, it also showed that girls felt less in control: for a higher proportion first sexual intercourse was under pressure (22 per cent for girls and 10 per cent for boys) and was more frequently regretted (41 per cent for girls compared with 22 per cent of boys).

There is plenty of evidence, however, that roles can be reversed and men can find themselves in the emotionally vulnerable position. In the Glasgow study some described themselves as being in love and trying to attract a partner: 'I've been in love but I've never been sort of – I'll say that she is, she is the one I've been looking for a long time...'. Moreover, in a study of 15–16 year old Londoners, young men ranked 'love' first and 'happiness' second when asked to list 'the most important things in life for you' (Brannen *et al.*, 1994: 71). Nevertheless, for young men to use the romantic discourse risks ridicule from conservative male peers for breaking with traditional norms.

Other influences on young people's sexuality

Social class

Age at first intercourse is still strongly influenced by social class in Britain. In the first NATSAL survey amongst 16–24 year olds the median age of first intercourse for those in Social Classes IV and V was 16 while for Social Class I it was 18 (Johnson *et al.*, 1994). Amongst 16–24 year olds in the second NATSAL, 21 per cent of non-manual respondents reported first intercourse before 16, whilst amongst manual workers 31 per cent of young men and 33 per cent of young women did so (Wellings *et al.*, 2001). In the SHARE study there were similar variations by social class at age 14 (Henderson *et al.*, 2002). At age 16 socioeconomic factors did not predict SHARE boys' sexual experience or condom use when other factors were taken into account, but for girls, owner occupation predicted both later sexual experience and more condom use, while father's higher social class predicted later sexual experience. See Appendix 2 for more detail on this.

Differing economic circumstances generate different perspectives on sex: deprived young people see fewer future alternatives to justify postponing sexual activity, using contraception consistently (Vanwesenbeeck *et al.*, 1999), or terminating a pregnancy if they conceive (Smith, 1993). Furthermore, social class strongly shapes culture, which involves values that perpetuate the status quo. Thus middle class teenagers tend to invest in skills of future value and defer sexual gratification, while deprived teenagers focus on improving their immediate social status through, for instance, fashion, sexiness and sexual experience (Thomson, 2000).

Education

Lower expectations for education and lower educational levels are associated with earlier onset of sexual activity (West *et al.*, 1993), lower rates of contraceptive use (West *et al.*, 1993; MacDowall *et al.*, 2002) and more unwanted pregnancies (Kiernan, 1995; Social Exclusion Unit, 1999). Educational level is clearly related to social class but both have been found to have independent effects (Johnson *et al.*, 1994), those of educational level being stronger (West *et al.*, 1993; Wellings *et al.*, 2001). The incentive to avoid early pregnancy seems to stem from having a stake in the future of an economically advanced society, for which educational aspirations and level seem to be a marker (UNICEF, 2001).

Ethnicity

Very little published research has been conducted on the sexual behaviour of ethnic minorities in Britain (Bradby and Williams, 1999), yet NATSAL indicates that ethnicity is at least as important a factor as social class. Age at first intercourse varies considerably between ethnic groups and shows pronounced gender differences: only 1 per cent of Pakistani and Bangladeshi women reported having had sex before the age of 16, compared with 8 per cent of white women and 10 per cent of black women (Johnson *et al.*, 1994); for men it is 11 per cent, 19 per cent and 26 per cent respectively.

The survey findings probably reflect the different meanings that sexual relationships have between ethnic groups, as discussed in Chapter 8.

Media

In some surveys young people's second most widely reported source of sexual information is the media (Todd *et al.*, 1999). Newspapers, magazines and television tend to reinforce gender stereotypes in their portrayal of young people's sexuality, presuming heterosexuality, depicting young men as always wanting sex and young women as interested in emotions (Batchelor and Kitzinger, 1999). Male magazines aim to titillate rather than educate while female magazines provide information and advice about sex. Thus the media tend to confirm the gendered understandings of sex learnt from same-sex friends.

Perhaps the most important influence of the popular media is their general portrayal of young people as sexually active, in romantic relationships, or seeking to be so (Cope-Farrar and Kunkel, 2002). This may contribute to young people's exaggerated impressions of others' sexual experience, and view that they themselves are inexperienced by comparison. In the SHARE study those with higher estimates of their peers' level of sexual activity were more likely to report having had sexual intercourse themselves. Although there has been virtually no research on the impact of the media on sexual behaviour in Britain, in America strong associations have been found between television exposure and higher sexual activity (Strasburger and Donnerstein, 1999).

Family

Social influences on young people's sexual behaviour seem to start in infancy, the emotional climate of one's family shaping one's interactional competence in intimate relationships (Vanwesenbeeck et al., 1999). A childhood characterised by emotional warmth, close contact, clarity of rules, predictability and respect of individuality is associated with more competent management of relationships and behaviour. Conversely, sexual or physical abuse in childhood can result in low self-esteem, depression and low assertiveness, all of which can contribute to self-destructive behaviour and reduced ability to set safe sexual limits (Vanwesenbeeck et al., 1999).

When young people are asked about their most important sources of information about sex, parents generally come well below friends, the media and school (Todd et al., 1999; Wellings et al., 2001). Yet there is now considerable quantitative evidence that both the structure of families and the processes within them are associated with young people's sexual behaviour (West and Sweeting, 2002; Sweeting et al., 1998). In the SHARE study, those with a younger mother, those who did not live with both biological parents and, in particular, those who were not living with either parent, were more likely to have sex at an early age, while young women with a younger mother were less likely to use condoms. Among 16 year olds who reported a high degree of parental monitoring, only 24 per cent reported having had sex, compared with 57 per cent of those who had a low degree of parental monitoring. A longitudinal analysis confirmed that the causal link is primarily (but not entirely) from parental monitoring to sexual behaviour (Wight et al., forthcoming). Weekly disposable income was not entirely attributable to parents, being a combination of pocket money and earnings, but it too was strongly related to age at first intercourse. (See Appendix 2 for more detail.)

Survey findings only provide crude indicators of the significance of young people's home life. The measures used are probably only proxies for more important aspects of family culture that need to be explored through qualitative research (for example, Brannen *et al.*, 1994). Nevertheless, these findings suggest that young people might overlook the influence of parents when they are asked how they learn about sex, not because parental influence is insignificant but because it is so pervasive.

Religion

Part of the influence of ethnicity is through religion: NATSAL found that for both sexes those with a non-Christian religion (for example, Muslims and Hindus) were the least likely to have had sex before the age of 16, while those who reported no religion were most likely (Johnson *et al.*, 1994). In Scotland the *degree* of religious belief has also been found to be strongly related to sexual behaviour (Henderson *et al.*, 2002; West *et al.*, 1993), and for young women, but not young men, greater religious belief is associated with greater condom use. However, Johnson *et al.* (1994) point out that there might also be some reverse causation: religious beliefs which do not support one's preferred pattern of behaviour might be allowed to lapse.

Interaction within relationships

The broad social factors discussed above all contribute to the heterogeneity of young people's sexual behaviour, but the interaction between sexual partners is also extremely important. For instance, at the start of a relationship both partners often strive to maintain ambiguity about their sexual intentions, in order to maintain their, or their partner's, dignity in case their wishes are not mutual (Kent *et al.*, 1990). Consequently the issue of condoms cannot be raised until it is almost inevitable that sexual intercourse will occur: usually at too late a stage to go and get one. Conversely, if one partner is explicit about his/her wish to have sex (which would be more likely within the predatory discourse) it transforms the interaction and allows for discussion of precautions.

This is illustrated in the SHARE data at age 16. Although there was some social patterning of young women's condom use, for both sexes it was characteristics of the sexual relationship that were most strongly correlated with condom use at first intercourse, the most important being whether or not sexual partners discussed taking precautions prior to having sex. This pattern is the same at 14 years (Henderson *et al.*, 2002). For young women, not expecting to have sex and being under pressure to do so made condom use less likely. For boys, having sex at an earlier age made it less likely. See Appendix 1 for more detail.

Conclusion

Although there is a tendency to identify typical behaviour when reviewing research findings on young people's sexual behaviour, this chapter has highlighted the diversity in their sexual attitudes and practices. While a tenth of 16–19 year olds reported having had sex at 14 or younger, another tenth had sex at 19 or not at all (Wellings *et al.*, 2001). By the age of 16 most people have not yet had sex, but 13 per cent of girls and 10 per cent of boys report three or more heterosexual partners.

The meanings that these relationships have also vary considerably, from romantic idealisation to boosting one's esteem with same-sex peers, both amongst young women and young men, although traditional gender roles still predominate. These conventional norms give young men greater power in sexual relationships, quite apart from their greater physical strength, and there is still evidence that some use this to pressure their partners into sex.

These variations are not surprising given the complex influences on young people's sexual behaviour. While social factors *associated* with sexual behaviour are readily identified – social class, educational level, family composition, ethnicity, parenting style – the *way* in which they are related is far more difficult to determine. Some factors (for example, educational level) might influence behaviour through expectations of the future, while others (for example, weekly disposable income) might be proxies for some other influence. What is clear is that the factors shaping young people's sexual behaviour stem from their childhood experiences, from social circumstances in their teens and from their expectations of the future.

Young people's sexual behaviour is particularly subject to moral censure, since many cultures perceive sex as an adult activity. Yet the sexual risk-taking that young people engage in is shared by older age groups as well. The differences are a matter of degree, and young people's use of contraception is actually more widespread than that of older age groups. Even the usually fraught nature of young people's early sexual experiences is, to some degree, revisited when entering new relationships as an adult.

What distinguishes young people's sexuality is the way initial heterosexual experiences are entered into with an understanding that is highly gender-specific, largely shaped through same-sex peer groups. As sex-segregation in friendship groups breaks down and experience of heterosexual relationships increases, young people gradually develop a greater understanding of the sexual beliefs and desires of the opposite sex.

There is only space here to identify some of the most important implications of these findings for policy and practice, some of which are addressed elsewhere in this book. Attempts to encourage more social integration between genders should be extended in order to promote a greater understanding, and, hopefully, greater respect, for the ways in which the opposite gender views sexual relationships (Wight *et al.*, 1998). Related to this are the benefits of encouraging more communication about sex between (potential) sexual partners, this being strongly associated with condom use. The diversity of young people's sexual experiences suggests that targeted sex education programmes should be developed to meet the needs of the particularly vulnerable minority who start sex in their early teens. However, more generally, the research evidence suggests that the best way to modify high-risk behaviour is to give young people long-term aspirations through educational and employment opportunities. Finally, parents' strong influence on their children's behaviour must be better understood and interventions developed to support them in their parenting roles.

References

Batchelor, S. and Kitzinger, J. (1999) *Teenage Sexuality in the Media*. Edinburgh: Health Education Board for Scotland.

Bradby, H. and Williams, R. (1999) Behaviours and expectations in relation to sexual intercourse among 18–20 year old Asian and non-Asians. *Sexually Transmitted Infections* **75**: 162–7.

Brannen, J., Dodd, K., Oakley, A. and Storey, P. (1994) *Young People, Health and Family Life*. Buckingham: Open University Press.

Cope-Farrar, K. M. and Kunkel, D. (2002) Sexual messages in teens' favorite prime-time television programs, in J. D. Brown, J. R. Steele and K. Walsh-Childers (eds) *Sexual Teens, Sexual Media: Investigating Media's Influence on Adolescent Sexuality*. New Jersey/London: Lawrence Erlbaum Associates.

Currie, C. and Todd, J. (1993) *Health Behaviours of Scottish Schoolchildren. Report 3: Sex Education, Personal Relationships, Sexual Behaviour and HIV/AIDS Knowledge and Attitudes*. Edinburgh: Health Education Board for Scotland and Research Unit in Health and Behavioural Change.

Gagnon, J. H. and Simon, W. (1974) *Sexual Conduct: The Social Sources of Human Sexuality*. London: Hutchinson.

Griffin, C. (1985) *Typical Girls? Young Women from School to the Job Market*. London: Routledge and Kegan Paul.

Henderson, M., Wight, D., Raab, G. M., Abraham, C., Buston, K., Hart, G. and Scott, S. (2002) Heterosexual risk behaviour among young teenagers in Scotland. *Journal of Adolescence* **25**: 483–94.

Holland, J., Ramazanoglu, C., Sharpe, S. and Thomson, R. (1998) *The Male in the Head: Young People, Heterosexuality and Power*. London: Tufnell Press.

Hollway, W. (1984) Gender difference and the production of subjectivity, in J. Henriques, W. Hollway, C. Urwin, C. Venn and V. Walkerdine (eds) *Changing the Subject: Psychology, Social Regulation and Subjectivity*. London: Methuen.

Information and Statistics Division Scotland (1998) Teenage pregnancy in Scotland 1987–1996. *Health Briefing no.98/01*. Edinburgh: ISD.

Irwin, C. and Millstein, S. (1986) Biopsychosocial correlates of risk-taking behaviors during adolescence. *Journal of Adolescent Health Care* **7**: 82S–96S.

Jakobsen, R. (1997) Stages of progression in noncoital sexual interactions among young adolescents: an application of the Mokken Scale Analysis. *International Journal of Behavioural Development* **21**(3): 537–53.

Johnson, A. M., Wadsworth, J., Wellings, K. and Field, J. (1994) *Sexual Attitudes and Lifestyles*. London: Blackwell Scientific.

Kent, V., Davies, M., Deverell, K. and Gottesman, S. (1990) Social interaction routines involved in heterosexual encounters: prelude to first intercourse. Paper presented at Fourth Conference on Social Aspects of AIDS, 7 April

1990, South Bank Polytechnic, London.

Kiernan, K. (1995) Transition to parenthood: young mothers, young fathers associated factors and later life experiences. *Welfare State Programme Discussion Paper 113*. London School of Economics.

MacDowall, W., Gerrassu, M., Nanchahal, K. and Wellings, K. (2002) *Analysis of Natsal 2000 Data for Scotland*. Edinburgh: Health Education Board for Scotland.

McRobbie, A. (2000) *Feminism and Youth Culture*. London: Macmillan.

Mirza, H. S. (1992) *Young, Female and Black*. London: Routledge.

Rhode, D. L. (1993) Adolescent pregnancy and public policy. *Political Science Quarterly* **108**: 635–69.

Schofield, G. (1994) *The Youngest Mothers*. Aldershot: Avebury.

Sharpe, S. (1985) *Just Like a Girl: How Girls Learn to be Women*. Harmondsworth: Penguin.

Smith, T. (1993) Influence of socioeconomic factors on attaining targets for reducing teenage pregnancies. *British Medical Journal* **306**: 1232–5.

Social Exclusion Unit (1999) *Teenage Pregnancy*. London: The Stationery Office.

Strasburger, V. C. and Donnerstein, E. (1999) Children, adolescents and the media: Medical and psychological impact. *Pediatrics* **103**: 129–39.

Sweeting, H., West, P., Richards, M. (1998) Teenage family life, lifestyles and life chances: associations with family structure, conflict with parents and joint family activity. *International Journal of Law, Policy and the Family* **12**: 15–46.

Tschann, J. M., Adler, N. E., Millstein, S. G., Gurvey, J. E. and Ellen, J. M. (2002) Relative power between sexual partners and condom use among adolescents. *Journal of Adolescent Health* **31**(1): 17–25 July.

Thomson, R. (2000) Dream on: the logic of sexual practice. *Journal of Youth Studies* **3**(4): 407–427.

Todd, J., Currie, C. and Smith, R. (1999) *Health Behaviours of Scottish Schoolchildren: Sexual Health in the 1990s*. Technical Report no. 2. Edinburgh: Research Unit in Health and Behavioural Change.

UNICEF (2001) A league table of teenage births in rich nations. *Innocenti Report Cards 3*, Florence, Italy: Innocenti Research Centre.

Vanwesenbeeck, I., van Zessen, G., Ingham, R., Jaramazovib, E. and Stevens, D. (1999) Factors and processes in heterosexual competence and risk: an integrated review of the evidence. *Psychology and Health* **14**(1): 25–50.

Wellings, K., Field, J., Johnson, A. M. and Wadsworth, J. (1994) *Sexual Behaviour in Britain*. London: Penguin.

Wellings, K. and Mitchell, K. (1998) Risks associated with early sexual activity and fertility, in J. Coleman and D. Roker (eds) *Teenage Sexuality: Health, Risk and Education*. Amsterdam: Harwood.

Wellings, K., Nanchahal, K., Macdowall, W., McManus, S., Erens, B., Mercer, C. H., Johnson, A. M., Copas, A. J., Korovessis, C., Fenton, K. A. and Field, J. (2001) Sexual behaviour in Britain: early heterosexual experience. *The Lancet* **358**:1843–50.

West, P. and Sweeting, H. (2002) A review of young people's health and health behaviours in Scotland. *Occasional Paper no. 10*. Glasgow: MRC Social and Public Health Sciences Unit.

West, P., Wight, D. and Macintyre, S. (1993) Heterosexual behaviour of eighteen year olds in the Glasgow area. *Journal of Adolescence* **16**(4): 367–96.

Wight, D. (1994) Boys' thoughts and talk about sex in a working class locality of Glasgow. *Sociological Review* **42**(4): 703–37.

Wight, D. (1996) Beyond the predatory male: the diversity of young Glaswegian men's discourses to describe heterosexual relationships, in L. Adkins and V. Merchant, *Sexualising the Social: Power and the Organisation of Sexuality*. London: Macmillan.

Wight, D., Abraham, C. and Scott, S. (1998) Towards a psycho-social theoretical framework for sexual health promotion. *Health Education Research: Theory and Practice* **13**(3): 317–30.

Wight, D., Henderson, M., Raab, G., Abraham, C., Buston, K., Scott, S. and Hart, G. (2000) Extent of regretted sexual intercourse among young teenagers in Scotland: a cross-sectional survey. *British Medical Journal* **320**, 6 May: 1243–44.

Wight, D., Raab, G., Henderson, M., Abraham, C., Buston, K., Hart, G. and Scott, S. (2002) The limits of teacher-delivered sex education: interim behavioural outcomes from a randomised trial. *British Medical Journal* **324**, 15 June: 1430–3.

Wight, D., Williamson, L. and Henderson, M. (forthcoming) article on parenting.

Appendix 1

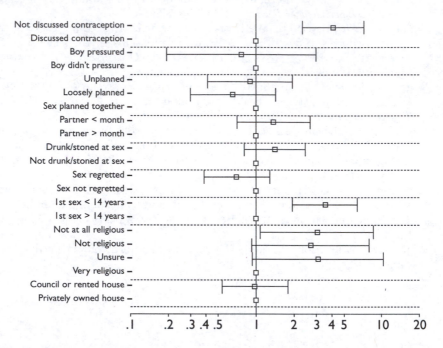

Figure 2A1.1 Factors associated with young men's reported non-use of condoms at first intercourse, by mean age 16 years, 1 month (SHARE data)

Note: Multivariate predictors: odds ratios relative to the baseline categories (on vertical line 1), with 95 % confidence intervals as horizontal bars (greater width = less precision; if crosses 1 not statistically significant).

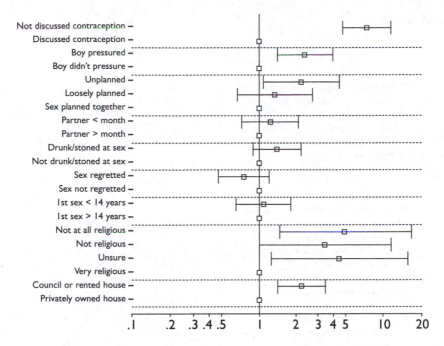

Figure 2A1.2 Factors associated with young women's reported non-use of condoms at first intercourse, by mean age 16 years, 1 month (SHARE data)

Note: Multivariate predictors: odds ratios relative to the baseline categories (on vertical line 1), with 95 % confidence intervals as horizontal bars (greater width = less precision; if crosses 1 not statistically significant).

Appendix 2

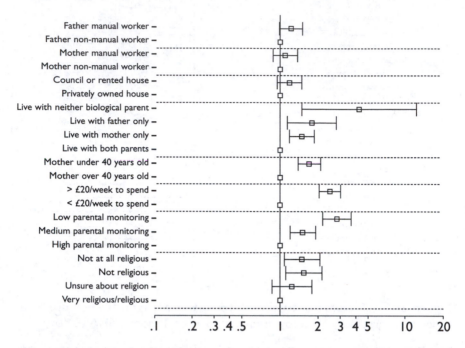

Figure 2A2.1 Factors associated with young men's reported sexual intercourse, by mean age 16 years, 1 month (SHARE data)

Note: Multivariate predictors: odds ratios relative to the baseline categories (on vertical line 1), with 95 % confidence intervals as horizontal bars (greater width = less precision; if crosses 1 not statistically significant).

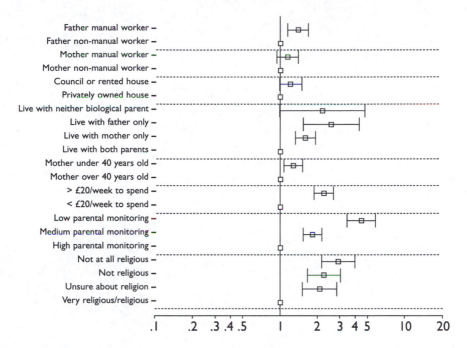

Figure 2A2.2 Factors associated with young women's reported sexual intercourse, by mean age 16 years, 1 month (SHARE data)

Note: Multivariate predictors: odds ratios relative to the baseline categories (on vertical line 1), with 95 % confidence intervals as horizontal bars (greater width = less precision; if crosses 1 not statistically significant).

Part Two

International and UK Policy Contexts

Why policy matters

National policies are key vehicles for framing issues, identifying priorities and allocating resources. They influence action at national, regional and local levels, encouraging and enabling work in some areas and making it more difficult for work in other areas. For example, in the UK the focus on teenage pregnancy in the past decade has led to a great deal of research and action focused on young women, potentially at the expense of young men.

Policy is undoubtedly influenced by the social, cultural and political context in which it is developed. It is 'a conscious contrivance ... in some sense a moral act' with 'a normative element at the heart' (Anderson, 1978: 20). Some issues on which there are strong divisions in social attitudes, or where developments are likely to be controversial, may be avoided or approached in a less direct way by policy makers concerned about public response. Conversely, policy, and the action that occurs as a result, may also shape public attitudes, setting the tone for more constructive debate and discussion and potentially shifting social norms. In reality, it is difficult to identify and distinguish between these upward and downward processes.

The focus of this section

The chapters in this section look at policies relating to sexual health in a range of countries. They explore the possible links between these policies and data showing evidence of need and effectiveness in relation to sexual health outcomes. Such comparisons 'can lead to fresh and exciting insights and a deeper understanding of issues that are of central concern in different countries' (Hantrais and Mangen, 1996: 3). Bearing in mind the above discussion about the development of policy, the effectiveness of policy is also determined by a range of factors which are difficult to substantiate, including local implementation, resource allocation, conflicting priorities and timeliness.

Over the last 20 years of research in social policy there has been a shift from large scale survey research with an emphasis on descriptive, culture-free approaches (Hantrais, 1999), to smaller scale, qualitative research more reliant on cultural sensitivity (Clasen, 1999). At the same time, policy makers increasingly have been looking to learn from and even 'borrow' policies from other countries, especially in light of moves towards evidence based policy making, as endorsed in the UK Modernising Government agenda (Davies *et al.*, 2000). Many policies in one country are now adapted from those shown to be promising in other countries, the UK Sure Start programme, for example, built directly on Head Start in the USA.

Of course there are problems in adapting policies from other countries. Health care systems, social welfare systems, legislation and social/cultural value systems differ, raising questions about whether policies devised in one national context can be applied elsewhere (Antal *et al.*, 1996; Hantrais and Mangen, 1996). Indeed, some suggest that since every culture has its own norms and values, it is impossible to apply policy lessons that have been learnt elsewhere (Antal *et al.*, 1996).

Even if applying a policy is in principle a good idea, practical differences between the source country and the borrowing country can significantly influence the relative effectiveness of implementation. For example, Sure Start is founded on evidence that early intervention improves outcomes for children across a wide range of indicators but it is also dependent on having enough professionals to deliver the programme in the way required to maximize effectiveness. In the UK some concerns have been expressed about whether there are sufficient health care staff to ensure this.

There are other difficulties when attempting to compare the impact of policies across different regions. Obtaining reliable data on sexual health is difficult and obtaining directly comparable data across countries is virtually impossible, especially when historical data are required. For example, administrative data on abortions have not been routinely recorded in Australia until recently, while STI rates are difficult to obtain in the USA due to the extent (and confidentiality) of private treatment. Another issue is that teenage births and abortions are presented as rates per 1000 women so in theory a reduction in teenage birth rates could arise from a real reduction in the actual number of births with a stable population or no change in actual numbers but an increase in population size within the relevant age group. Finally, lack of availability of trend data makes measuring changes over time difficult.

Another challenge is in relation to interpreting data changes over time, since separating the impact of policy changes from that of broader social changes is very difficult. For example, a teenage birth 30 years ago had quite different social and cultural significance from today and this is likely to have had an impact on rates of teenage pregnancy and parenthood.

So policy comparison requires an acute awareness of how cultural and political contexts influence policy development. It also requires care in interpreting cause and effect, given difficulties in making direct links between policy implementation and actual impact. Despite this, and even where policies cannot directly be borrowed, for example because they conform to different norms, these chapters show that elements may be adapted or built on, extending the range of options from which policy makers may choose with regard to improving sexual health.

References

Anderson, C. W. (1978) The logic of public problems: evaluation in comparative policy research, in E. A. Douglas (ed.), *Comparing Public Policies: New Concepts and Methods*. Beverly Hills: Sage.

Antal, A., Dierkes, M. and Weiler, H. N. (1996) Cross-national policy research: traditions, achievements and challenges, in A. Inkeles and M. Sasaki, *Comparing Nations and Cultures: Readings in a Cross-Disciplinary Perspective*. New Jersey: Prentice-Hall.

Clasen, J. (1999) *Comparative Social Policy: Concepts, Theories and Methods*. Oxford: Blackwell.

Davies, H. T. O., Nutley, S. and Smith, P. C. (2000) *What Works? Evidence-Based Policy and Practice in Public Services*. Bristol: Policy Press.

Hantrais, L. (1999) Comparing family policies in Europe, in J. Clasen (ed.), *Comparative Social Policy: Concepts, Theories and Methods*. Oxford: Blackwell.

Hantrais, L. and Mangen, S. (1996) *Cross-National Research Methods in the Social Sciences*. London: Pinter.

3 Policy Developments in the United Kingdom

ELIZABETH BURTNEY, DEIRDRE FULLERTON and ALISON HOSIE

Key issues

- Different data collection systems, particularly in the area of conceptions and births, make it difficult to draw accurate comparisons across the four countries.
- There are inconsistencies in sexual health policy and service provision across the UK, which result in differing patterns of sexual health outcomes.
- However, the positive moves that have been initiated at national and local levels to address sexual health in a holistic manner should be recognized.

Overview

This chapter presents a broad picture of policy approaches towards the promotion of teenage sexual health in the United Kingdom, providing detail where possible on the four individual countries' (England, Scotland, Northern Ireland and Wales) approaches to sexual health. However, there are instances where it is not possible to include Northern Ireland mostly because of data collection issues, and where this is the case, Britain will be used instead of the UK to cover England, Scotland and Wales. It does not draw conclusions about the likely impact of policy in the UK context, rather it serves to set the context and bring the reader up to date with recent and current policy and focus around sexual health.

Introduction

During the 1960s and 1970s Britain (rather than the UK) was actually a pioneer with regard to developments in sexual health policy (Hosie, 2001). However British society is now generally viewed as having more conservative views with regard to sex and sexuality (Hofstede, 1998; Jones et al., 1985).

While other European responses in the 1980s to growing concerns around sexual health including HIV were more pragmatic, British responses were more based on moral judgements, as reflected in both the way in which popular press now reports on sexual health matters (Batchelor *et al.*, forthcoming) and in the policy focus on teenage mothers. Despite recent moves to tackle existing inequity (for example, the repeal of clause 2A in Scotland, Section 28 in England and Wales) and poor sexual health, Great Britain now has the highest rates of teenage pregnancies in Western Europe and has recently witnessed a substantial rise in sexually transmitted infections (STIs).

Subsequent chapters in this book describe policies elsewhere in Europe and other English speaking countries. This chapter is devoted to presenting the current sexual health picture in the UK and outlining policy which has been established, both historically and more recently, to respond to the sexual health needs of young people in particular.

Sexual health in the UK

Pregnancy, birth and abortion

The UK has one of the highest rates of teenage pregnancies in the developed world, second only to the USA and almost five times higher than the Netherlands (UNICEF, 2001). The rates over the last 20 years in the UK have actually remained relatively unchanged at the same time as most of Western and Northern Europe witnessed a decline in rates through the 1980s and 1990s.

However, there are indications in England and Scotland of a downward trend. For example, the conception rate among under 18 year olds for 2001 is 3.5 per cent lower than in 2000, and is 10 per cent below the 1998 rate (TPU, 2003). The likely outcome of teenage conception is also changing, with a slight increase in rate of terminations, particularly among older teenagers (TPU, 2003; ISD Scotland, 2003).

There is evidence of variations between and within the four UK countries. For example, Wales has consistently had a higher conception rate than England: 68.5 per 1000 15–19 year olds compared with 62.2 in England (ONS, 1999). However, presenting pregnancy and outcome information across the four countries is difficult since data are not collected consistently and services available in the different regions vary. For example, pregnancy and abortion rates are reported for different age groups in the four countries. In England and Wales pregnancy rates are reported for under 18 year olds, whereas in Scotland data are presented for 13–19 year olds. In addition, miscarriages are recorded in a variety of ways so conception rates are also difficult to compare. Therefore the tables which follow are presented on a country by country basis allowing for these differences.

It should be noted that there are particular issues pertinent to Northern Ireland as the 1967 Abortion Act does not apply. The grounds for termination in Northern Ireland are very strict, and termination is provided only if the pregnancy poses an immediate threat to a woman's life. This

Table 3.1 Pregnancy* and outcome data for England, 2001

	Total conceptions	Conception rates	Percentage leading to legal abortion
Under 16s	7 396	7.9 (based on 13–15 population size)	55.9
Under 18s	38 439	42.3 (based on 15–17 population size)	46.0

Note: *The data for conception statistics in England and Wales are compiled by combining information from registration of births and notifications of legal abortions. They do not include miscarriages or illegal abortions.

Table 3.2 Birth rate and abortion data for Northern Ireland, 2001

	Total live births	Live birth rate	Total legal abortions performed in England to NI teenagers
15–19 years	1 527	23	319

Table 3.3 Pregnancy* and outcome data for Scotland, 2001

	Total conceptions	Conception rates	Percentage leading to legal abortion
13–15 years	728	7.9	52.7
16–19 years	8 785	70.6	41.2
13–17 years	4 098		

Note: *Data in Scotland are based on information on the number and rate of pregnancies in young women under the age of 20, including cases based on maternities (pregnancies ending in live or still-birth) and pregnancies resulting in a therapeutic abortion or miscarriage which required hospital inpatient or day-case treatment.

Table 3.4 Pregnancy* and outcome data for Wales, 2001

	Total conceptions	Conception rates	Percentage leading to legal abortion
15–19 years	5 800	62.9	Not available

Note: *Calculated on the same basis as English data.

compares with the remainder of the UK, where abortion is permitted for medical as well as sociomedical or social reasons including low income, poor housing, young or old age, and having a certain number of children (Ketting, 1993). Women residing in Northern Ireland requiring a termination of pregnancy must access private services in England and Wales, and limited information is available on how many avail themselves of these services, since statistics are based on the addresses they give, which may be false or local to the service.

Across the UK there is a link between area deprivation and teenage pregnancy and parenthood. For example, English electoral wards with the highest levels of deprivation also have teenage pregnancy rates higher than the national average. In Northumberland, a large county in northern England, pregnancy rates varied from 19.7 per 1000 under 18 years in a ward ranked 199th most deprived in the country (Tynedale) to 70.6 per 1000 under 18 years in the 17th most deprived ward in the country (Wansbeck) (DETR, 2001; ONS, 2001). Similar patterns emerge in Scotland and Northern Ireland (FPA NI, 2003a; ISD Scotland, 2003). Outcome of pregnancy is also linked to socioeconomic status, with young women from areas of higher deprivation opting for birth rather than termination (ISD Scotland, 1998).

While deprivation is strongly associated with teenage pregnancy and parenthood, other factors include a history of generational teenage pregnancy in the family, low education attainment, having been 'looked after' by local authorities, and having been abused (SEU, 1999; Fullerton, 2002). Chapter 2 presents a more detailed analysis of these factors.

Sexually transmitted infections (STIs)

STIs are an increasing cause of morbidity among young people (aged 16–25) and rising rates among younger teenagers are a particular cause for concern (PHLS, 2002, Nicoll *et al.*, 1999). Sexually active young people are at increased risk of STIs as they are more likely to have higher numbers of sexual partners and have more concurrent partners (Wellings *et al.*, 2001; Johnson *et al.*, 2001). This is compounded by the influence of alcohol and drugs on sexual behaviour among teenagers (SEU, 1999; Cooper, 2002). Young people who are intoxicated are more likely to engage in risky sex (Testa, 1997; Wechsler *et al.*, 1994).

There is evidence that condom use is improving, with eight out of ten 16–19 year olds reporting condom use at first intercourse in Britain and fewer than one in ten teenagers reporting unprotected sex at first intercourse. However, a rise in the number of reported partners may offset some of the public health benefits of increased condom use (Wellings *et al.*, 2001).

Since 1996, rates of genital chlamydial diagnoses in GUM clinics have increased disproportionately in young people (Figure 3.1). During 2002, rates among males were highest in those aged 20–24 years (837/100,000), whereas

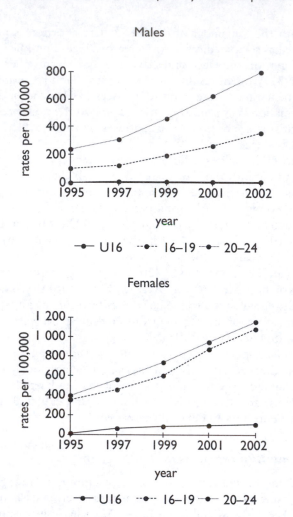

Figure 3.1 Diagnoses of uncomplicated genital chlamydial infection in UK GUM clinics by sex and age group, 1995–2002*

Note: Data unavailable for Scotland 2000, 2001 and 2002 at time of press
Source: www.hpa.org.uk/infections/topics_az/hiv_and_sti/epidemiology/sti_data.htm

in females they were highest in 16–19 year olds (1,201/100,000). Overall, 1.2 per cent of 16–19 year old females in England, Wales and Northern Ireland had a diagnosis of chlamydia in a GUM clinic in 2002. Whilst it is likely that the rise in chlamydial diagnoses reflects increased uptake of testing for chlamydia as a result of improved public and professional awareness of the infection and improved testing technologies, the current statistics are likely to underestimate the real rate of infection as chlamydia is symptomless in many cases.

Findings from the recent pilot projects in England have indicated that the incidence of chlamydia may be particularly high among young women, as approximately 10 per cent of women under the age of 25 attending health care settings in the Wirral were found to be infected with chlamydia (PHLS, 2002). The most recent NATSAL study also indicated an increasing incidence of chlamydia, with one in 45 men and one in 66 women involved in the survey being infected with chlamydia. This rose to one in 33 for 18–24 year olds. The research found that nearly all people carrying the infection were unaware of it (Fenton *et al.*, 2001).

HIV infection

Between 1982 and 2002 there were a total of 56,108 new HIV infections diagnosed in the UK. The number of new infections has increased per year since 1994, partly explained by an increase in reporting and diagnosis. It is estimated that there are currently 33,500 people living with HIV, of whom 9400 have not yet had their HIV status diagnosed (PHLS, 2002).

Of particular interest are routes of HIV transmission. A dramatic decline occurred in transmission between injecting drug users in the early 1990s when needle exchange programmes became widely accessible. Moreover, while originally transmission was predominantly via sex between men, the main source of transmission currently is through heterosexual contact, with many people becoming infected abroad. Policy has started to look at prevention measures aimed at heterosexual adults, in particular travellers abroad (DoH, 2001; Scottish Executive, 2001).

HIV is uncommon among young heterosexual people in the UK (PHLS, 2002). Among young sexually active people in the UK, homosexual young men are at greater risk, and heterosexual teenagers with STI infections are at a higher risk of acquiring HIV if they have an HIV infected partner (HPA, 2003).

Table 3.5 HIV infected individuals by year of diagnosis

Probable route of infection	1992 or earlier	1995	1998	2000	2002 *	Total 1992–2002
Sex between men	14 422	1 465	1 352	1 488	1 481	29 322
Sex between men and women	3 035	850	1 158	1 981	2 899	17 870
Injecting drug use	2 492	183	130	108	84	3 954
Other	2 277	147	170	243	874	4 962
Total	22 226	2 645	2 810	3 820	5 338	56 108

Note: *provisional figures at time of press
Source: CDR, 2003

Sexual activity

The most recent National Survey of Sexual Attitudes and Lifestyles (NATSAL) reported that the median age at which young people first have sexual intercourse in Britain has fallen from 21 for women and 20 for men born in the early 1930s (Johnson *et al.*, 1994) to 16 for both sexes born in the early 1980s (Wellings *et al.*, 2001). The proportion of the 2000 sample reporting first intercourse before 16 years was 30 per cent for men and 26 per cent for women (Wellings *et al.*, 2001). The proportion of women who reported first intercourse before 16 years increased up to, but not after, the mid-1990s.

Alongside this there has been a sustained increase in condom use at first intercourse and a decline in the number of both men and women reporting no contraceptive use at first intercourse with decreasing age at interview. Factors associated with sexual activity and contraception use are discussed in Chapter 2.

Northern Ireland was not included in the NATSAL survey. However, in a recent survey of sexual attitudes and lifestyles of young people in Northern Ireland, 37 per cent of respondents reported sexual intercourse before the age of 17, and 27 per cent had sex before the age of 16. A quarter of respondents failed to use any protection at first intercourse (FPA NI/ University of Ulster, 2002).

Policy and legislative frameworks

Human rights and sexual rights

The human rights agenda has a significant impact on many aspects of sexual health, in particular access to information, education and services. The United Nations Convention on the Rights of the Child (UN General Assembly, 1989) states that young people have a right to express their views on matters affecting them and that these views should be given due weight. In addition, it is the right of the child to seek information and support to inform their decisions. This has particular relevance for school-based sex education where there can be conflict between the wishes of the parent and child.

While sexual rights are not stated in law, the World Health Organization has stated that:

Sexual rights ... include the right of all persons, free of coercion, discrimination and violence to:
- the highest attainable standard of health in relation to sexuality, including access to sexual and reproductive health care services
- seek, receive and impart information in relation to sexuality
- sexuality education
- respect for bodily integrity

- choice of partner
- decide to be sexually active or not
- consensual sexual relations
- consensual marriage
- decide whether or not, and when to have children
- pursue a satisfying, safe and pleasurable sexual life.

(World Health Organization, 2002)

Development of sexual health policy across the UK

In 1967 the Abortion Law Reform Act entered the statute books, a ground-breaking piece of legislation which would impact upon the whole of Europe over the decades to follow. Contraception in many forms had been available in Britain since the early twentieth century but it was not legally sanctioned until 1967. Under Section 1 of the National Health Service (Family Planning) Act in 1967, a duty was placed on health authorities to provide contraceptive services to all who requested them and then in 1968, the FPA (formerly the Family Planning Association) changed its policy to allow unmarried women the right to have access to contraceptive services (Hosie, 2001). By 1970, all health clinics were legally obliged to provide contraceptive services to all who requested them across the UK, apart from Northern Ireland where the Abortion Law did not apply. This continues to be the case and abortion services are not accessible in Northern Ireland although the FPA Northern Ireland is currently lobbying to rectify this inequity (FPA NI, 2003b).

In 1974, family planning clinics previously run by the FPA were taken over and run by the NHS and as a result, local authorities were obliged to provide contraceptive services and contraceptives free of charge. For example, a Family Planning Circular produced by the Scottish Home and Health Department stated that 'family planning services should be available to all who need them and ... should be so organized as to avoid any bar to the provision of services to the unmarried' (Bury, 1984: 37); no mention was made in this or prior documentation about any restriction of the age at which these services could/could not be provided. Then in 1983 emergency contraception was made legally available in Britain, and was widely advertised by organizations such as Brook and the FPA.

In 1983 Victoria Gillick brought a test case against her health authority to prevent doctors prescribing contraception to under-16s without parental consent; this was to have serious implications for the sexual health of young people in Britain. The first ruling was made in favour of the rights of young people under 16 to access contraception without parental consent but this was overturned in 1984, only to finally be overturned again, in favour of young people's rights, by the House of Lords in 1985. Whilst this case technically only affected English law, it has had ramifications for the provision of contraception to young people in other parts of the UK. Following this case the Fraser Guidelines were developed to help advise medical professionals about young people and their health rights; from this developed the 'Gillick competence-test'. This test is expected to be used by all medical professionals faced with a decision over whether to prescribe contraception to young women under the legal age of consent.

In Northern Ireland the legal age of consent is 17 but the medical age of consent is 16, as for the rest of the UK. A doctor or health professional can provide contraceptive advice or treatment without parental consent but they must try to obtain the young person's consent to involve his or her parents before providing treatment (FPA NI, 2001).

While there was a focus on developing policy around services, sexual health promotion was ongoing, and most active in response to the arrival of HIV and AIDS. Following the discovery of HIV, the ban on advertising condoms commercially was lifted in 1987, which was followed by a large number of government and non-government funded HIV and sexual health promotion activities. The first large HIV media campaign was launched in 1986 and ran until the end of 1987. This was followed by almost annual campaigns running until the end of 1993. Media work was supported by community initiatives and local health promotion activity focusing on HIV prevention and monies for sexual health were mainly directed at HIV. Towards the mid-1990s, practitioners were moving towards more integrated sexual health work and were creative in directing monies ring-fenced for HIV towards broader sexual health promotion initiatives.

Current sexual health policy

Since the mid-1990s, and in particular since devolution from Westminster in the late 1990s, a number of important developments both in policy and government attitudes to teenage sexual health have had an impact on the promotion of teenage sexual health. For example, an increased awareness at both national and local level of the need to base sexual health provisions for young people on the actual needs and contexts of young people's lives led to a more holistic approach (Hosie, 2001).

Table 3.6 summarizes the most recent sexual health policies across England, Scotland, Northern Ireland and Wales. In short, Scotland and Wales built policies around 'sexual health' rather than specific issues such as teenage pregnancy, while England and Northern Ireland instead adopted separate strategies on sexual health and teenage pregnancy.

In its two-pronged approach, England first developed a teenage pregnancy strategy with a comprehensive and wide-reaching action plan incorporating media campaigns, work with parents, sex and relationships education and a focus on teenage parents, both male and female. This was followed by a sexual health and HIV strategy, focusing more on service development. In Scotland, initial targets were around teenage pregnancy, set within a broad context, for example through funding of community wide initiatives like *Healthy Respect* (Scottish Office, 1999). However, more recent policy development has focused on enhancing sexual health at a population level. Wales, drawing on work from England, produced a sexual health strategy with emphasis on education and service provision while reflecting on the importance of the broader societal context. Finally, Northern Ireland followed a similar path to England, firstly producing a teenage pregnancy strategy followed by the current development of a sexual health strategy. Major differences between England and Northern Ireland include budget levels and approaches. Northern Ireland has a tradition for cross-department working, in part facilitated by the structure of government, and this is reflected in its teenage pregnancy work which cuts across housing, education, social services and health in a more meaningful way.

Teenage pregnancy and parenthood

Teenage pregnancy is worth considering separately because of the level of policy interest, especially since 1992 with the launch of *The Health of the Nation* (DoH, 1992) and its target to reduce the rate of pregnancy to under-16s by 9.4 per 1000 in 1989 to 4.8 per 1000 by the year 2000. These targets were adopted to a certain extent by the other countries, and work to achieve them was supported by an increase in the number of places where young people could access sexual health services. This development continued for a period of about five years from 1992, and coincided with the only noted decline in teenage pregnancy rates over the last two decades (Hadley, 1998).

In England, the Social Exclusion Unit teenage pregnancy report and action plan (SEU, 1999) is now the key policy document in this area. The report was initially criticized for its sole focus on teenage pregnancy as research supported the need for integrated sexual health promotion messages and approaches and there were concerns about 'unjoined-up thinking'. However, it has also been cited as an example of good practice in applying a well researched, multi-faceted approach to health promotion to a specific issue with young people (House of Commons, 2002/2003).

The large evidence base in relation to teenage pregnancy and the breadth of factors influencing decisions relating to this aspect of sexual health provided a legitimate argument for addressing this vast issue alone. A sole focus on teenage pregnancy also provided the opportunity to take a long-term developmental approach from early years through to adulthood, advocating a cross-departmental approach. Since the publication of the *Teenage Pregnancy Strategy* in 1999 the rate of conceptions to young women aged under 18 has decreased by 10 per cent (Independent Advisory Group, 2003).

Table 3.6 Related sexual health policies in England, Scotland, Northern Ireland and Wales

Related policies	Advantages and disadvantages	Key aims and targets (where specified)
England *National teenage pregnancy strategy*	• Joined up approach supported by widespread consultation. • Strong evidence base. • Substantial budget attached. • An independent advisory group and external evaluation planned from outset. • Short and long term targets. • Criticized for sole focus on teenage pregnancy rather than broader sexual health. • £60 million cross deparmental budget.	**Aims** • Reduce the rate of teenage conception. • Increase participation of teenage parents in education, training or employment to reduce long term risk of social exclusion. **Specific targets** • Halve the rate of conceptions among under 18 year olds in England by 2010 (with an interim reduction target of 15% by 2004 included in NHS Plan) • Increase the participation of teenage mothers in education, training or work to 60% by 2010 to reduce the risk of long term social exclusion.
Better prevention, better services, better sexual health: The national strategy for sexual health and HIV	• Seeks to address inequalities of access. • Tiered approach to service provision. • Strong evidence base. • Additional investment of £47.5 million over first two years of strategy life. • Clear recommendations for practice and research.	**Aims** • Reduce the transmission of HIV and STIs. • Reduce the prevalence of undiagnosed HIV and STIs. • Reduce unintended pregnancy rates. • Improve health and social care for people living with HIV. • Reduce the stigma associated with HIV and AIDS.

Table 3.6 continued

Related policies	Advantages and disadvantages	Key aims and targets (where specified)
England (continued)		
Better prevention, better services, better sexual health: The national strategy for sexual health and HIV (continued)	• Little linkage with TP strategy. • Medical model rather than social, reflected in recommendations. • Little attention to contraceptive education/services.	**Specific targets:** • Reduce by 25% the number of newly acquired HIV infections and gonorrhoea infections by the end of 2007. • All GUM clinic attendees should be offered an HIV test on their first screening. • Increase the uptake of the test by those offered it to 40% by the end of 2004 and to 60% by the end of 2007. • Reduce by 50% the number of previously undiagnosed HIV infected people attending GUM clinics who remain unaware of their infection after their visit by the end of 2007. • Increase uptake of hepatitis B vaccine by the end of 2003; all homosexual and bisexual men attending GUM clinics should be offered hepatitis B immunization at their first visit. • Increase uptake of the first dose of the vaccine, in those not previously immunized, to 80% by the end of 2004 and 90% by the end of 2006.

Table 3.6 continued

Related policies	Advantages and disadvantages	Key aims and targets (where specified)
England (continued)		
Better prevention, better services, better sexual health: The national strategy for sexual health and HIV (continued)		**Specific targets** • Increase uptake of the three doses of vaccine, in those not previously immunized, within one of the recommended regimens, to 50% by the end of 2004 and 70% by the end of 2006. (Strategy supported by a broadbased action plan to improve services, information and support, reduce inequalities in sexual health and improve health, sexual health and wellbeing.)
Northern Ireland		
Teenage pregnancy and parenthood: strategy and action plan	• Clear links made to social inequalities • Holistic approach to interventions. • Provides pointers to good practice aimed at preventing unintended teenage pregnancies. • Implementation budget identified. • Wide consultation process. • Little linkage to local level strategies.	**Aims** • Facilitate a reduction in the number of unplanned births to teenage mothers. • Minimize the adverse consequences of those births to teenage parents and their children. **Specific targets** • Reduce by 20% the rate of births to teenage mothers by 2007

Table 3.6 continued

Related policies	Advantages and disadvantages	Key aims and targets (where specified)

Northern Ireland (continued)

| *Teenage pregnancy and parenthood: strategy and action plan (continued)* | | **Specific targets:**
• Reduce by 40% the rate of births to teenage mothers under 17.
• 75% of teenagers should not have experienced sexual intercourse by the age of 16.
• 100% of teenage mothers of compulsory school age should complete formal education.
• 50% of teenage mothers should participate in post 16 education beyond school leaving age. |
| There is also a sexual health strategy under development. | | |

Scotland

| *Report of the HIV Health Promotion Strategy Review Group* | • Multidisciplinary group.
• Broad approach to HIV prevention beyond clinical approaches.
• Clear evidence base.
• Specific action for series of groups in need of additional support. | The remit of the group was to review the effectiveness of current HIV/AID health promotion activities and consider change in emphasis of activity and funding. Concluded that health boards and other agencies need to revisit current approaches to prevention in an effort to progress from the current 'steady state' to downward track in number of new infections. |

Table 3.6 continued

Related policies	Advantages and disadvantages	Key aims and targets (where specified)
Scotland (continued)		
Report of the HIV Health Promotion Strategy Review Group (continued)	• Limited impact as recommendations to review funding rather than coming with funding attached.	Report highlights a series of recommendations aimed at specific population groups including gay men, adult heterosexual population, young people and injecting drug users.
Enhancing Sexual Wellbeing in Scotland: A Sexual Health and Relationships Strategy		**Aims and targets of the draft strategy** • To influence the cultural and social factors that impact on sexual health. • To support everyone in Scotland to acquire and maintain the knowledge, skills and values necessary for sexual wellbeing. • To improve the quality, range, consistency, accessibility and integration of sexual health services. The draft strategy recommends that the Scottish Executive retains their target for reducing teenage pregnancy, that is to achieve a 20% reduction in the 13–15 year old age group between 1995 and 2010. In addition the draft strategy recommends that this should be complemented by other targets to provide a more comprehensive picture of sexual health.

Table 3.6 continued

Related policies	Advantages and disadvantages	Key aims and targets (where specified)
Wales		
Strategic framework for promoting sexual health in Wales	• Integrated approach. • Strong evidence base for recommendations. • Wide representation on reference group. • Emphasis on education and health promotion as well as clinical support. • Action Plan included as part of consultation. • No budget.	**Aims** • Improve the sexual health of the population of Wales. • Enhance the general health and emotional wellbeing of the population by enabling and supporting fulfilling sexual relationships. **Targets** None stated but aims supported by series of more detailed objectives and comprehensive action plan to support the aims.

Similar to England, Northern Ireland has also focused on teenage pregnancy, identifying it as one of the four priorities within the Promoting Social Inclusion initiative (DHSSPS, 1999) and a strategy to reduce teenage pregnancies and support teenage parents (DHSSPS, 2002). While neither Wales nor Scotland has specific strategies for teenage pregnancy and parenthood, a reduction of teenage conceptions is among the aims of the sexual health strategies in Wales (National Assembly for Wales, 2000) and a target of 20 per cent reduction in the 13–15 year old group between 1995 and 2010 was set in Scotland (Scottish Office, 1999). The draft Scottish sexual health strategy recommends the Scottish Executive retain their target for reducing teenage pregnancy but shoud ensure other targets are introduced to provide a more comprehensive picture of sexual wellbeing. (Scottish Executive, 2003)

Age of consent and sexual conduct

In England, Scotland and Wales the age of consent was equalized in 2000 for heterosexual and homosexual sex to 16 years, while in Northern Ireland it is 17 years.

In recent years, there has been some ambiguity regarding the reality of this legislation for teenagers aged 12–15 who both consent to sexual intercourse. Interpretation varies between professionals. For example, while in most cases teachers who are aware of a pupil having sex before 16 years are duty bound to act on this information (as it becomes a child protection issue), for health professionals there is a greater element of individual judgment. In England the Sexual Offences Bill proposed in 2003 has the potential to criminalize underage sex between consenting teenagers, with a maximum five-year sentence applicable.

Sex and relationships education

Chapter 11 describes in detail the situation across the UK in terms of school-based sex and relationships education (SRE). While SRE started from a base of inconsistency in terms of quality and quantity across different schools, there have been major steps in improving the quality of provision. Steps taken include the production of guidance for staff involved in the delivery of SRE, guidance for parents on the role of SRE, the inclusion of SRE in school inspections in England, Scotland and Wales, and increased attention to the evidence base for school-based sex education. Furthermore, SRE has become embedded in a whole school approach through the Health Promoting School concept (Scotland and Northern Ireland) and the National Healthy School standard (England and Wales). These offer the potential to act as unifying models for those promoting health (Young and Williams, 1989), and may help raise the health profile and provide scope for schools to consider the formal as well as hidden curriculum. This is of particular importance for sexual health, where factors beyond those directly associated with sex, for example self-esteem, are as important as those directly associated.

Sexual health services

Across the UK, health boards have a duty to ensure that young people have access to holistic health services – including sexual health services – that meet their needs. However, interpretation of what constitutes appropriate services varies between providers. Some areas offer specific services directed at the needs of young people, for example Brook Clinics and Caledonia Youth in Scotland. Others rely on mainstream services, which often do not meet the needs of young people (Hosie, 2001, 2002a). For young people in particular, the importance of confidentiality, anonymity, ease of geographic access, appropriate opening times, suitable location and premises and, arguably most important, the attitudes of staff, has been noted (Hosie, 2001; Hosie and Silver, 2001). If these factors are not considered, and young people are unable to access services they feel appropriate, they may be prevented from using contraception within their sexual relationship. Research exploring the issue of sexual health service provisions internationally has documented that the ease of access to services is crucial to their use by young people (CRD NHS, 1997; Fullerton *et al.*, 1997; Hadley, 1998; Liinamo *et al.*, 1997; Peckham, 1993; Zabin *et al.*, 1986).

There is growing awareness of the need to provide services for young people at policy level, for example the English sexual health strategy has earmarked funding for pilot projects in primary care youth services to target young people. However, in some areas this has met with resistance, for example in Northern Ireland the FPA and Brook are regularly targeted by religious groups who picket outside the premises.

The importance of the link between SRE and service provision has been highlighted (House of Commons, 2003; Kirby, 2001; Vincent and Dod, 1989), and policy makers are responding to this through for example the development of the role of the school nurse. In some parts of the UK the school nurse provides input to the SRE and may also support this with an onsite service. There are political and moral issues surrounding this work which have still to be resolved by both national and local level players (see Chapter 4 for further discussion of the role of school nurses).

Support for teenage parents

Increasingly policy is recognizing the need to include work with pregnant teenagers and young mothers as part of the prevention cycle. As described in Chapter 2, there is evidence to suggest that young women who themselves had teenage mothers are more likely to have an early pregnancy. In addition, the education and employment opportunities often missed by young mothers make poverty more likely, which again influences early sex and pregnancy. The Teenage Pregnancy Strategy (1999) in England and the Teenage Pregnancy and Parenthood Strategy (2002) in Northern Ireland have explicit aims of supporting teenage mothers to continue and/or re-enter education or employment, and there are growing examples of initiatives to facilitate this work. In 2001 the DfES in England published guidance for schools on the education of school age parents (DfES, 2001) and through the Standards Fund established reintegration officers and specialist units to support young parents continue with their education (Hosie, 2002b). In addition, extra childcare and support through Connexions and Sure Start Plus are just some examples of the different initiatives aimed at supporting young parents and their children.

However, it remains difficult for young parents in society as there is still stigma associated with teenage parenthood. For example, the notion that young women get pregnant in order to benefit financially is still rife but unsupported by evidence. But it is the case that while parenthood is seldom 'planned', often adequate precautions to avoid it are not taken, and this in part is linked to the fact that parenthood is not an unattractive option for some young women. Turner (2001) suggested that 'the fewer the opportunities that a young woman has, the less motherhood is viewed as problematic' (Turner, 2001: 309), and that rather than the fewer opportunities being viewed as a reason to conceive, 'once pregnant, the reasons for avoiding motherhood [as opposed to abortion] may seem less significant' (Turner, 2001: 310). Indeed, a number of studies show that while girls would have delayed pregnancy given the choice, the positive benefits of motherhood, including reconnection with education and a greater sense of purpose, were overwhelming (Selman *et al.*, 2001; Hosie, 2002b).

Conclusion

Sexual health in the UK is of increasing concern, reflected through policy development across the four countries. Focus is moving from a narrowly defined prevention approach to a more holistic social model reflecting the growing evidence which links broader socioeconomic factors to sexual health. However, while the policy is moving in a similar direction, the resource to back any policy change is not consistent. England has invested heavily in both the Teenage Pregnancy Strategy and the Sexual Health and HIV Strategy, which does not appear to be the case in Wales or Northern Ireland. It is not yet clear what budget will be available in Scotland. This in part can be explained by resources available; however, clear financial investment is more likely to facilitate better working on the ground and subsequently better outcomes.

While policy and resources are important to improve sexual health, cultural change is also required and this seems to be falling behind the pace of policy change. For example, the repeal of clause 2A in Scotland was met by overwhelming media attention and public outcry from some corners. Stories from tabloid press still carry headlines that condemn teenage sex. This is compounded by the inability to separate developing sexuality from sexual intercourse. Indeed, this moral stance in relation to teenagers is broader than the media, and can be viewed in the very policy documents that set out to improve the situation. For example, the foreword to the teenage pregnancy report (SEU, 1999) from the Prime Minister talks about our 'shameful record' of teenage pregnancies rather than taking a more positive stance to the promotion of sexual health and wellbeing of young people. If sexual health is to be improved in the UK, attitudes will need to move from this condemning position to be more accepting of teenage sexuality.

References

Batchelor, S., Kitzinger, J. and Burtney, E. (forthcoming) *Representing Young People's Sexuality in the 'Youth' Media*. Health Education Research.

Bury, J. K. (1984) *Teenage Pregnancy in Britain*. London: Birth Control Trust.

Cooper, M. L. (2002) Alcohol use and risky sexual behavior among college students and youth: evaluating the evidence. *Journal of Studies on Alcohol* **64**: 101–17.

CRD NHS (1997) Prevention and reducing the adverse effects of unintended teenage pregnancies. *Effective Healthcare Bulletin* **3**(1).

CDR (2003) *Weekly* 4 September 2003.

DETR (2001) Deprivation Ranks: *Indices of Deprivation 2000: District Level Presentations*.

DfES (2001) *Guidance on the Education of School Age Parents*. London: Stationery Office.

Department of Health (1992) *Health of the Nation: A Strategy for Health in England* (Cmnd. 1986). London: HMSO.

Department of Health (2001) *Better Prevention, Better Services, Better Sexual Health. The National Strategy for Sexual Health and HIV*. London: Department of Health.

Department of Health, Social Services and Public Safety (1999) *Promoting Social Inclusion Initiative*. Belfast: DHSSPS.

Department of Health, Social Services and Public Safety (2002) *Teenage Pregnancy and Parenthood: Strategy and Action Plan 2002–2007*. Belfast: DHSSPS.

Fenton, K. *et al.* (2001) Sexual behaviour in Britain: reported sexually transmitted infections and prevalent genital Chlamydia trachomatis infection. *British Medical Journal* **358** Dec 1: 1851–4.

FPA NI (2001) The legal position regarding contraceptive advice and provision to young people, *FPA NI Factsheet*. Belfast: FPA NI.

FPA NI (2003a) Teenage Pregnancy. *FPA NI Factsheet*. Belfast: FPA NI.

FPA NI (2003b) Abortion. *FPA NI Factsheet*. Belfast: FPA NI.

FPA NI, University of Ulster (2002) *Towards Better Sexual Health: A Survey of Sexual Attitudes and Lifestyles of Young People in Northern Ireland*. London: FPA.

Fullerton, D. (2002) Preventing and reducing the adverse effects of unintended teenage pregnancy, in E. Burtney, *Teenage Sexuality: Evidence into Action*. Scotland: Edinburgh Health Education Board.

Fullerton, D., Dickson, R. and Sheldon, T. (1997) Preventing and reducing the adverse effects of teenage pregnancy. *Health Visitor* **70**(5): 197–9.

Hadley, A. (1998) *Getting Real: Improving Teenage Sexual Health*. Fabian Society. London: College Hill Press.

Health Protection Agency (2003) http://www.hpa.org.uk/infections/topics_az/hiv_and_sti/hiv/general.htm#who

Hofstede, G. (and associates) (1998) *Masculinity and Femininity: The Taboo Dimension of National Cultures.* London: Sage.

Hosie, A. (2001) *A Comparative Exploration of Social Policy Relating to Teenage Pregnancy in Finland and Scotland.* Unpublished doctoral thesis, Stirling University.

Hosie, A. (2002a) *Evidence into Action: Sexual Health Policy Analysis In Selected European Countries.* Edinburgh: HEBS.

Hosie, A. (2002b) Teenage Pregnancy in Young Women of School Age: an exploration of disengagement from the education system. *Society for the Study of Social Problems Annual Conference*, Chicago, 15–17 August 2002.

Hosie, A. and Silver, C. (2001) Overcoming the first hurdle: young people and access to sexual health services in Scotland, England, Finland and the Netherlands. *Helsinki: European Population Conference*, 7–9 June 2001.

House of Commons Health Committee (2003) *Sexual Health: Third Report of Session 2002/2003* **1.** London: HMSO.

Independent Advisory Group (2003) Independent Advisory Group on Teenage Pregnancy: *Annual Report 2002–2003*, Teenage Pregnancy Unit, London: Stationery Office.

Information and Statistics Division Scotland (1998) Teenage pregnancy in Scotland, 1987–1996. *Health Briefing*, 98/01: 1–7. Edinburgh: ISD.

Information and Statistics Division Scotland (2003) http://www.isdscotland.org

Johnson, A. M., Wadsworth, J., Wellings, K. and Field, J. (1994) *Sexual Attitudes and Lifestyles.* London: Blackwell Scientific.

Johnson, A., Mercer, C. M., Erens, B., Copas, A. J., McManus, B., Wellings, K. *et al.* (2001) Sexual behaviour in Britain: partnerships, practices and HIV risk practices. *Lancet* **358**:1835–52.

Jones, E. F., Forrest, J. D., Goldman, N., Henshaw, S. K., Lincoln, R., Rosoff, J. I., Westoff, C. F. and Wulf, D. (1985) Teenage pregnancy in developed countries: determinants and policy implications. *Family Planning Perspectives* **17**: 53–63.

Ketting, E. (1993) Abortion in Europe: current status and major issues. *Planned Parenthood in Europe* **22**: 4–6.

Kirby, D. (2001) *Emerging Answers: Research Findings on Programs to Reduce Unwanted Teenage Pregnancy.* Washington DC: National Campaign to Prevent Teenage Pregnancy.

Liinamo, A. *et al.* (1997) Taking adolescents seriously: four areas of Finland, in A. Hardon and E. Hayes, *Reproductive Rights in Practice: A Feminist Report on the Quality of Care.* London: Zed.

National Assembly for Wales (2000) *A Strategic Framework for Promoting Sexual Health in Wales.* Cardiff: Health Promotion Division.

Nicoll, A., Catchpole, M., Cliffe, S., Simms, I. and Thomas, D. (1999) Sexual health of teenagers in England and Wales: an analysis of national data. *BMJ* **318**: 1321–2.

Office of National Statistics (ONS) (1999) Conceptions: age of woman at conception, England and Wales. (Personal communication: data awaiting publication).

ONS (2001) Conception rates. *Population Trends* **103**, Spring 2001; Report: 86–112.

Peckham, S. (1993) Preventing unintended teenage pregnancies. *Public Health* **107**: 123–33.

Public Health Laboratory Services (PHLS) (2002) *Sexual Health in Britain. Recent Changes in High Risk Sexual Behaviours and the Epidemiology of Sexually Transmitted Infections Including HIV.* London: PHLS. www.phls.org.uk.

PHLS, DHSSPS, and the Scottish ISD Collaborative Group (2001) *Sexually Transmitted Infections in the UK: New Episodes Seen in Genitourinary Medicine Clinics 1995–2000. Trends in Sexually Transmitted Infections with Special Reference to Young People.* London: PHLS.

Scottish Executive (2003) *Enhancing Sexual Wellbeing in Scotland: A Sexual Health and Relationships Strategy.* Scottish Executive, Edinburgh.

Scottish Executive Health Department (2001) *Report of the HIV Health Promotion Strategy Review Group.* Edinburgh: Stationery Office.

Scottish Office (1999) *Towards a Healthier Scotland.* Edinburgh: Stationery Office.

Selman, P., Richardson, D., Speak, S. and Hosie, A. (2001) *Monitoring of the DfES Standard Fund Grant: Teenage Pregnancy.* University of Newcastle, Newcastle upon Tyne.

Social Exclusion Unit (1999) *Teenage Pregnancy.* London: Stationery Office.

Teenage Pregnancy Unit (2003)
http://www.info.doh.gov.uk/tpu/tpu.nsf

Testa, M. (1997) Alcohol and risky sexual behavior: event-based analyses among a sample of high-risk women. *Psychology and Addictive Behaviour* **11**: 190–210.

Turner, K. M. (2001) *Predictable Pathways? An Exploration of Young Women's Perceptions of Teenage Pregnancy and Early Motherhood.* Unpublished Doctoral Thesis, University of Stirling.

UNICEF (2001) A league table of teenage births in rich nations, *Innocenti Report Card No. 3.* Florence, Italy: UNICEF Innocenti Research Centre

UN General Assembly (1989) *United Nations Convention on the Rights of the Child.*

Vincent, M. and Dod, P. (1989) Community and school based interventions in teen pregnancy prevention. *Theory into Practice* **28**: 191–7.

Wechsler, H., Davenport, A., Dowdall, G., Moeykens, B. and Castillo, S. (1994) Health behavioral consequences of binge drinking in college: a national survey of students on 140 campuses. *Journal of the American Medical Association* **272**:1672–7.

Wellings, K., Nanchal, K., Macdowall, W., McManus, S., Erens, B., Mercer, C. *et al.* (2001) Sexual behaviour in Britain: early heterosexual experience. *The Lancet* **358**: 1843–50.

World Health Organization (2002) Technical consultation on sexual health. www.who.int/reproductive-health/gender/sexual_health.html#4

Young, I. and Williams, T. (1989) *The Healthy School.* Scottish Health Education Group/World Health Organization Regional Office for Europe.

Zabin, L. S., Hirsch, M. B., Smith, E. A. *et al.* (1986) Evaluation of a pregnancy prevention programme for urban teenagers. *Family Planning Perspectives* **18**(3): 119–26.

4 Sexual Health Policies and Trends in Europe

ALISON HOSIE

> **Key issues**
>
> - There is no 'magic bullet' policy solution to the successful promotion of young people's sexual health; awareness of the variety of policies that can impact upon young people's lives and their sexual behaviour is needed.
> - Whilst social attitudes towards sex and sexuality are a reflection of normative values, they are not fixed. Social policy can be used as a tool to reflect and facilitate positive attitudinal change.
> - Young people face similar situations and have to make similar decisions about their sexual behaviour; many European countries offer positive examples of how to support them in making those choices safely.

Overview

This chapter presents a broad picture of policy approaches towards the promotion of teenage sexual health across Europe, as well as a more focused analysis of Finland and the Netherlands. It examines the extent to which differences in social policy may be related to variation in a range of outcomes relating to teenage sexual behaviour.

Introduction

In order to explore different countries' approaches to the promotion of young people's sexual health, this chapter compares a variety of indicators related to the sexual health of young people. These include more common direct measures of sexual health but also some indirect indicators relating, for example, to education, which may be an important independent influence on sexual health outcomes (Hosie, 2001, 2002). There are significant issues outlined elsewhere regarding data availability and comparability, and regarding differences in cultural contexts and their impact on policy development and effectiveness, and it is difficult to make clear links between factors. However, the chapter will attempt to consider these links and to draw out implications for future policy development.

Overview of teenage sexual health indicators
Pregnancy, birth and abortion

The most common sexual health indicators explored are the rates of pregnancy, birth and abortion to young women, with live births providing the most accurate indicator as not all countries provide accurate abortion data (David, 1992). Figure 4.1 presents a combination of data on births and abortions to young women, to provide an approximated rate of pregnancy in a selection of countries.

Since longitudinal data are a better background against which to explore policy developments, Figure 4.2 presents the trends in rates of live births, for a selection of European countries. Trends vary but fit the general patterns found among other European countries: across Scandinavian and Nordic countries such as Finland and in West European countries such as France and

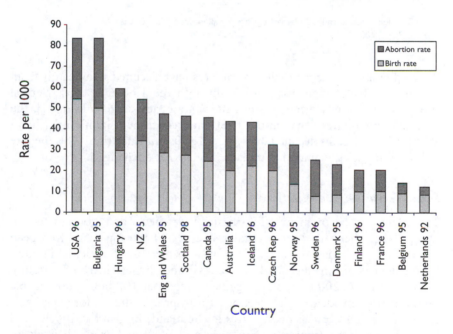

Figure 4.1 Rates of births and abortions to young women aged 15–19 in selected European countries, 1996 (or latest available year)

Note: Data for Scotland and the Netherlands are for all women younger than 20. Abortion data for Romania and France are only 80 per cent accurate.
Sources: ISD Scotland, 2000a and Singh and Darroch, 2000

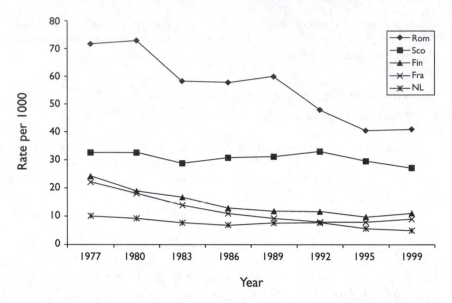

Figure 4.2 Trends in live birth rates per 1000 women aged 15–19 in selected European countries, 1977–99

Note: Data for Scotland and the Netherlands are for all women younger than 20
Source: Hosie, 2002

the Netherlands (except Britain), birth rates have declined significantly from the mid-1970s, though more slowly through the 1990s. In most Central and East European (former Eastern Bloc) countries, such as Romania, the decline in birth rates began in the 1980s and continued significantly thereafter. In Britain, rates declined during the 1970s but since the 1980s the rate of births to young women has remained relatively unchanged.

Sexually transmitted infections

The silent nature of many STIs means that they often go undetected. Despite this, there has been a notable rise in STI rates in many European countries over the last decade. This may be as a result of an actual increase in incidence or an increased awareness and hence increased testing (Panchaud *et al.*, 2000). Table 4.1 presents rates per 100,000 young people of gonorrhoea incidence in a selection of European countries for which data are available. This reveals higher rates for Scotland, England and Wales and Romania than for countries in Northern and Western Europe. It is worth noting that whilst the rate for young people in Scotland is notably higher than most European countries, it is considerably closer to those countries than to England and Wales combined and has a much more equal balance of incidence between men and women.

Table 4.1 Rates of gonorrhoea per 100,000 young people aged 16–19 in selected European countries, by gender

Country	Total	Rate per 100,000 Female	Male
Belgium (1996)	0.6	1.0	0.3
Denmark (1995)	5.0	5.0	5.0
England and Wales (1996)	76.9	95.7	59.1
Finland (1996)	3.7	3.8	3.6
France (1996)	7.7	8.4	7.0
Netherlands (1995)	7.7	7.5	7.8
Norway (1995)	6.7	9.1	4.4
Romania (1994)	65.8	U	U
Scotland (1998/9)	24.2	27.8	24.3
Sweden (1995)	1.8	2.0	1.5

Note: U = unavailable data
Sources: ISD Scotland, 2000b; Panchaud et al., 2000

Sexual activity and contraceptive use

Two large international studies conducted during the 1980s (Jones *et al.*, 1985; UN, 1988), revealed that in most European countries, the average age of first intercourse for young people was 17 years, and 16 in Northern Europe. A more recent study by Wellings *et al.* (1994) showed that differences between the age of initiation for young British and Scandinavian women were disappearing. Ross and Wyatt (2000) in the WHO study of health behaviour of school children confirmed that the proportions of Finnish and Scottish young women reporting first intercourse by age 15 (approximately 30 per cent) were almost identical.

The increased availability and more effective use of contraception helps to explain the dramatic fall in pregnancy rates during the 1970s across many European countries (Thompson, 1976; Yarrow, 1978).

While young people in Britain become sexually active at a slightly younger age than those in Western Europe, the difference is too small to account for the overall difference in rates of teenage pregnancy. It may be related to the fact that young people from many Northern and Western Europe are more likely to use reliable contraception (over 85 per cent) at first and subsequent intercourse than in Britain or Central–East European countries (below 55 per cent) (Ross and Wyatt, 2000; Hosie, 2002).

Policy relating to teenage sexual health promotion

School-based sex education

Over the last half century, the development of sex education in Europe has varied greatly (Papp, 1997), approaches to provision contrasting primarily as a result of differently weighted policy debates surrounding teenage pregnancy and abortion rates (Kosunen, 1996). Across most Western and Northern European countries, concern has been focused on the health consequences of early sexual activity (Davis, 1989; Kosunen, 1996), leading to the development of sex education based on positive sexual health promotion. In countries such as Britain and the USA, a moralistic stance on teenage sexual activity has lead to more restricted sex education aimed at preventing teenage sexual activity (Hosie, 2001). Figure 4.3 shows access levels in the mid-1990s across Europe.

Vilar's (1994) review revealed that despite a large proportion of European countries introducing some form of sex education into the curriculum by the mid-1990s, only Belgium, the Netherlands and the Nordic countries were classed as having provision adequately meeting the sex educational needs of young people (that is, providing information beyond the basics of sexual reproduction, pregnancy and contraception from a positive sexual health promotion stance). The remaining countries were classed as having inadequate education focusing primarily on the negative outcomes rather than on positive sexual health.

Sexual health services

In many European countries, young people can access sexual health services through a variety of mainstream providers. However, young people have many additional needs, which are often not met by provisions set up for use

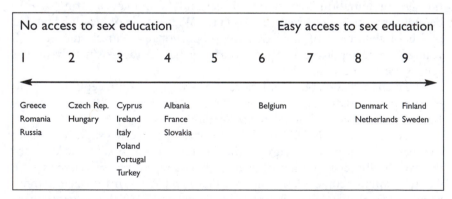

Figure 4.3 Access to school-based sex education in selected European countries

Source: Vilar, 1994: 11

by the whole population. International research exploring the issue of sexual health service provisions has shown that the ease of access to services is crucial to their use by young people (Zabin *et al.*, 1986; McIlwaine, 1994; Fullerton *et al.*, 1997; Liinamo *et al.*, 1997; NHS CRD, 1997; Hadley, 1998; Hosie and Silver, 2001). Confidentiality, opening times, visibility of a service (to parents/family), friendly services, positive professional attitudes are all key factors in young people's willingness and perceived ability to access sexual health services (FPA, 1994; Clements *et al.*, 1997; Liinamo *et al.*, 1997; Nelson, 1997; Hadley, 1998; Aggleton *et al.*, 1999; Cheesbrough *et al.*, 1999; SEU, 1999; Hosie and Silver, 2001; Turner, 2001).

Evidence from Europe and the USA supports the promotion of youth-specific clinics and school-based clinics. Jones *et al.* (1985, 1986) in a study of 37 industrialized nations, showed that specialized youth clinics which were fully integrated advice centres and linked to schools, were likely to be the most effective in promoting young people's sexual health, a view supported by Zabin *et al.* (1986), Allen (1991), Fullerton *et al.* (1997) and Hosie and Silver (2001). Services set up specifically for use by young people have been developed in countries such as Denmark, England and Wales, Finland, Germany, the Netherlands, Norway, Scotland, Sweden and Switzerland (Peckham, 1993; Kane and Wellings, 1999; Hosie, 2001). The extent to which this type of service has been developed, and its impact on young people's sexual health, however, varies between countries. For example, in England during the early 1990s there was a period of development of youth clinics which was reported to be well received and used by young people (Bloxham *et al.*, 1999). The main expansion of such services between 1990 and 1995 was followed by the first decline in pregnancy rates in ten years (Hadley, 1998). They were, however, not universally provided across the country resulting in a lack of equality of access for young people. Those most noted as likely non-attendees were 'younger teenagers, young men and those living in areas of deprivation for whom the motivation to avoid pregnancy may be undermined by high levels of unemployment' (Hadley, 1998: 14).

Education

Educational attainment and aspiration may play an important indirect role in the promotion of the sexual health of young people, in the desire to both delay parenthood and protect their health against STIs (Selman and Glendinning, 1996; SEU, 1999; Hosie, 2001, 2002). There are links between higher levels of educational attainment and higher levels of sexual knowledge (Kontula and Rimpelä, 1988), a higher age of first intercourse (Kane and Wellings, 1999), a higher age of first birth (Beets, 1999a, 1999b) and more effective contraceptive use (Hofmann, 1984; Morrison, 1985). Moreover, a significant relationship exists between higher stay-on rates at school aged 16–18 and lower teenage pregnancy rates in Europe (Hosie, 2001).

Although it is plausible to argue that rates of employment (or unemployment) among young people have a bearing on young people's willingness to remain in education, there are no significant links between rates of young people remaining in school across Europe and the rates of youth unemployment (aged 15–25) or rates of employment amongst women aged 15 and over (Hosie, 2001). This strengthens the theory that young people are remaining at school for reasons other than a lack of immediate employment prospects – for example, because of aspirations to achieve more educationally, which are unlikely to include the desire to become a parent at a young age.

In Britain there has been a strong drive in recent years to increase the proportion of young people in education to levels found in other European countries. The Department for Education and Skills *Public Service Agreement* (2002) in England seeks to have 90 per cent of young people completing a full-time programme enabling entry into higher education or skilled employment by the age of 22, and reiterates a previous government aim to increase participation in higher education to 50 per cent of those aged 18 to 30 by 2010.

Figure 4.4 presents the proportions of young people remaining in education aged 16–18, in a selection of countries and the comparatively low stay-on rates in Britain do not bode well for the targets described above.

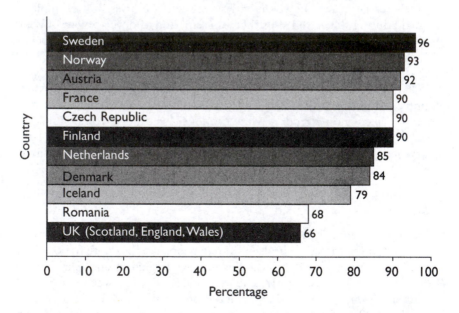

Figure 4.4 Percentage of young people in education aged 16–18 in selected European countries

Note: * = for Romania and the Czech Republic age grouping is 16–17; for the Netherlands age grouping is 17–18

Source: EC/Eurydice/Eurostat, 2000

Sexual health promotion in the Netherlands

It is often assumed that the Netherlands has always been a sexually 'liberal' country. However, prior to the 1960s, abortion and family planning were regarded as 'immoral practice', contraception was seen as the route to promiscuity (Ketting and Schnabel, 1980: 385) and sex education was viewed as 'a necessary evil at best' (Röling, 1993: 236) and was rarely provided in schools (Silver, 1999).

Faced with increasing birth rates to young women under 20 through the 1960s, peaking at 19.8 per 1000 women aged under 20 in 1967, the response was what Silver describes as a 'cultural trait of seeking practical solutions to social problems' (Silver, 1998: 8). Silver (1999) describes the Netherlands, with a mix of Catholics, Protestants and a large Jewish community, as a country where pragmatism and tolerance have developed out of necessity. Therefore, rather than a policy response aimed at preventing sexual activity amongst young people, the Dutch 'considered [it] more appropriate and effective to equip young people with the means to control the potential consequences of their sexual behaviour' (Silver, 1999: 17).

Since the nineteenth century Dutch sex legislation has applied two age limits, with 'sexual contacts' (without abuse or force) absolutely prohibited before the age of 12 and totally permissible from the age of 16. In the 'shady' area between 12 and 16, sexual contacts are punishable only when a complaint is lodged (http://www.ageofconsent.com/netherlands.htm). In 1991 the Dutch sex legislation was modernized whereby only the young person or their parents are allowed to bring charges. The fact that a young person is allowed to file charges is 'as unique as it is important. The new act sets great store on the young person's personal view of volition' (http://www.ageofconsent.com/netherlands.htm). Most importantly, it allows young people to report abuse without the presence of a parent/guardian or adult, who may well be the abuser, and it allows young people aged over 12 to obtain confidential information regarding sexual health and contraception if they need it.

School-based sex education

Although no statutory obligation to provide school-based sex education existed until 1993, there was widespread support and acceptance of sex education in schools from the early 1970s. Sex education was developed based on individual school needs, with an overall philosophy that sex is not taboo but rather it is a normal aspect of life and therefore sex education 'is integrated into the whole learning experience process and is treated like any other topic' (Silver, 1998: 26).

The majority of sex education is provided through the medium of biology, although the content and focus is generally very broad, with topics ranging from physical and mental maturation, growing up, puberty, menstruation, masturbation, relationships and love, sexuality, homosexuality, human reproduction, contraception, conception, pregnancy, miscarriage, abortion, birth, STIs and sexual abuse (Sheldon, 1997, 1998; Silver, 1998). Teaching environments and methods vary but generally teachers make use of both single and mixed-sex arenas and role-play is commonly used to promote communication and negotiation skills (Sheldon, 1997, 1998).

Sexual health services

The rigorous promotion of contraception to young people began in the early 1970s, aided by the development of the Rutgers Stichting Institute in 1969, which created venues for young people confidentially to access contraception and advice. This early promotion to young people differs from other countries such as Britain where the promotion of contraception to young people still attracts much negative attention. As early as 1974, soon after contraception became available to young people, the proportion of young people aged 16–20 using contraception was 86 per cent (Ketting and Schnabel, 1980), considerably higher than many European countries in the late 1990s (Ross and Wyatt, 2000). Additionally, although abortion technically remained illegal until 1985, by 1973 abortion clinics were widely accessible to all women. At the present time all women who are Dutch residents are entitled to abortions, which are funded by the government if performed in the country's abortion clinics. National health insurance or private insurance will cover the fees for abortions performed in hospitals (Pryor, 2001).

General education system and stay-on rates

The Netherlands has a very flexible system educational system, which does not restrict young people to one type or level of education. Secondary school begins at the age of 12 and can last for a period of five to eight years (full- and/or part-time). There are three main streams of secondary education that provide a basic three-year period from which pupils would either progress to general or vocational upper secondary education (de Bruijn and Howieson, 1995).

The Dutch system appears quite complicated with its varying streams; however, it offers choice for young people whereby entry into one particular stream does not mean confinement to that stream for the rest of their school career. Young people are encouraged to re-sit levels or move streams rather than to leave school, with little noted stigma for mixed age classes (Hosie, 2002). The stay-on rate post-16 in the Netherlands remains high until the age of 17 (90 per cent), at which point the percentage decreases by approximately 10 per cent per year group (EC/Eurydice/Eurostat, 2000).

The past two generations have witnessed a strong trend of women delaying parenthood and remaining in education for longer (Beets, 1999a). Silver (in Hosie, 2002) notes that being a young parent in the Netherlands is heavily stigmatized by young people themselves as life aspirations seem to act as behaviour regulators (Silver, 1998). Young people and adults in the Netherlands are not saying that young people do not have the right to be sexually active; rather that if they are, they should use contraception. This compares with views presented by the adult community in Britain, where there is emphasis on preventing sexual activity because it is perceived to be wrong for young people to have sex, rather than helping young people to delay or practise safer sex.

Sexual health indicators

Despite the more 'liberal' approach to teenage sexual health promotion in the Netherlands, and an age of sexual consent lower than most Western European countries, not only is the age of first intercourse amongst young people in the Netherlands a year older (17.5 years) than the rest of Northern and Western Europe (Francis, 1984) but 50 per cent of young women are already using oral contraceptives prior to first intercourse (Francis, 1994). In addition the 'Double-Dutch' combination of concurrent use of condoms and contraceptive pill to promote pregnancy and STI prevention has been well received among young people (Rademakers, 1991; Silver, 1998), which implies that effective contraceptive use is both well internalized and normalized amongst Dutch young people.

Figure 4.5 outlines the trend in live births to Dutch women under 20 years of age from 1966–99. Abortion rates are not available over this time period, but are acknowledged to have remained low since the early 1970s,

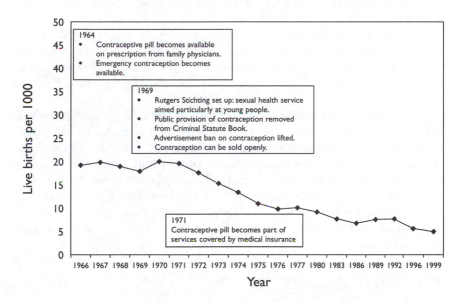

Figure 4.5 Time line of live births per 1000 women under 20 in the Netherlands

Source: EC/Eurydice/Eurostat, 2000

most recent data showing a rate of 4.0 per 1000 women under 20 (Hosie and Silver, 2001).

The reported incidence of syphilis (1.0 per 100,000) and gonorrhoea (7.7 per 100,000) among young people is very low (although there are reliability problems with these data) and although breakdown by age is not readily available in the Netherlands, the incidence of HIV at the end of 1999 was low in European terms, estimated at 15,000 of the whole population (Panchaud et al., 2000; EuroHIV, 2000).

Sexual health promotion in Finland

Finland is often subsumed under the Nordic banner in relation to sexual health policy. However, this has sometimes meant that important differences between Finland and other Nordic countries are overlooked. For example, it is often assumed that Finland has always had more 'liberal' sexual attitudes (Hosie, 2001), but prior to the 1960s sex was considered a very private issue (Väestöliittö, 1994). It was not until a noted rise in unwanted births and STIs during the 1960s that there was recognition for the need for policy change.

The first major policy change was to the abortion law, which prior to 1970 was only available under specified medical conditions (Väestöliittö, 1994). The 1970 law included two important new grounds, particularly for young women. First, social grounds for abortion were legitimized, and second, if a woman was under 17 at the point of conception, this in itself was considered grounds and needed only one rather than two doctors' permission (Hosie, 2001).

This was followed by the Public Health Act (1972), which placed a statutory obligation on municipalities (equivalent to local authorities in Britain) to provide free access to general health services, including all sexual health services (irrespective of age) and school health services (Kosunen and Rimpelä, 1996).

In the early 1970s the Finnish Penal Code set the legal age of heterosexual consent at age 16. However, this regulation was not intended to criminalize consensual sexual relationships between young people. Therefore, although the age of consent is set at 16, sexual relations between young people under the age of 16 are not considered as sexual abuse of children/young people if 'there is little difference in age or mental and physical maturity of the parties concerned' (http://www.ageofconsent.com/finland.htm). In practice therefore, if the sex is consensual and both parties are aged 14–15 years of age, sexual relations are not prosecuted (Hosie, 2001).

School-based sex education

Sex education was formally brought into the school curriculum in 1976, to help address the problem that the sexual health of young people was not improving in line with the rest of the population (Hosie, 2001). It was not taught as a separate subject; rather, the 'promotion of healthy sex and sexuality' (Hosie, 2001: 181) was contained within a range of compulsory curriculum subjects (Table 4.2). The National Board of Education (NBE) stipulated for all curriculum subjects, including those containing elements of sex education, what teachers should provide in terms of content, minimum timetabling and preferred methods for teaching, including an emphasis on active-learning based methods in single and mixed-sex classes. In this way, young people across the country had equal access to similar sex education.

Through the three grades the content of each class complemented what was being taught in each class from different perspectives, topics included: physical and emotional changes, menstruation, wet dreams, masturbation, dating, experimentation, pornography, respect and responsibility, trust, sexual relations, mutual consent, rape, pregnancy, contraception, prevention of STIs and HIV, abortion, alternate sexualities and preferences (NBE, 1998).

School health services and other provisions

The introduction of sex education was complemented by the development of a school health service, which provided every school in Finland with an on-site school health clinic. A school nurse was available on average 3–5 days, for young people to visit whenever they needed to (Hosie, 2001). Some nurses could also dispense contraception (based on municipal decisions) but where this was not possible young women were using the school nurse to arrange an appointment (Kosunen, 2000) to gain contraception from a municipal centre (Liinamo, 2000).

Table 4.2 Provision of sex education in Finland

Curriculum subject	Location of sex education	Teaching perspective	Hours of teaching	Teaching environment
Biology	Biological reproduction	Biological	Minimum 3, average 7 hours over 7–9th grades (12–16 yrs)	Mixed sexed
Home economics	Family education	Legal, social and ethical	1 hr/week 9th grade (14–16 yrs)	Mixed sexed
Physical education	Health education	Sexual health	1 hr/week 8th grade (13–15 yrs)	Single sexed

Source: Hosie, 2001

In 1983 a target was set to reduce abortions to young women under 20 by 7 per cent per annum, reflecting government concern not so much with young women becoming pregnant but rather with unintended and preventable pregnancies.

In 1987 the magazine *Sexteen*, which provides information about all aspects of sexual health and a sample condom, was sent to 16 year olds on their birthday (from 2001 at the request of young people the age was lowered to 15) (Hosie, 2001). Readership of this magazine is associated with higher levels of sexual knowledge (Liinamo, 2000). Also in 1987 emergency contraception was legalized, providing a further reproductive option.

By the late 1980s, in addition to municipal health centres and school health services, young people could also access non-governmental organization (NGO) youth clinics, providing a wide variety of access to contraception and advice about sexual health.

However, cutbacks were introduced within the provision of school health care in 1994, which has had two resulting impacts on school nursing. First, there was a change in the style of nurse training, with a move from youth specific for school nurses to general nursing for a geographical area, therefore reducing the number of school nurses trained to work with young people. Second, the workload and number of schools expected to be covered by one nurse increased in many areas, resulting in less time available to each school. In 1998 the National Board of Education had only just begun to realize the potential impact this could have on young people's sexual health, but already had growing concerns about how this was already impacting on the mental health of young people (Hosie, 2001).

General education system and stay-on rates

Educational reforms of 1972 developed a comprehensive school (*Perusk-oulu*) system that has been actively promoting the normality of continued education for young people beyond the compulsory level, which ends at age 16 (and is viewed as the 'prep' stage before the 'real' education begins), until at least the age of 19 (Hosie, 2001). All young people progress to undertake at least three years of further study (although approximately 5–8 per cent drop out annually) at either a vocational school or a high school. Alternatively, when young people's grades are not sufficient to continue at the school they wish, there is an opportunity to take a tenth year to improve their grades before continuing (Hosie, 2001).

As in the Netherlands, this system has helped to cultivate expectations and motivations for young people that may promote delaying pregnancy and parenthood and thereby contribute to improved sexual health outcomes.

In 1994 a new curriculum for the *Peruskoulu* devolved more decision-making powers to schools, reducing the number of compulsory subject hours and increasing optional hours. Two of the compulsory hours removed were one hour per week of physical education (health education) and home economics (family education). In 1994, cutbacks were also made in funding for school health services, resulting in considerably less school nursing time within individual schools (Hosie, 2001).

Sexual health indicators

Finnish researchers have argued that the development of more 'liberal' and pragmatic direct and indirect policies to promote teenage sexual health in Finland have not encouraged more young people to begin their sexual lives earlier (Kosunen and Rimpelä, 1996). Three studies into teenage sexual behaviour undertaken in 1986, 1988 and 1992 found similar rates of first intercourse among young women (30 per cent by age 15) and decreasing rates among young men (30–19 per cent by age 15) (Kosunen, 1993). The same studies revealed both an increase of contraceptive use at first intercourse and a decrease in proportions reporting no contraception with each survey (Kosunen, 1993).

Further to this, with available data on STIs considered to be over 70 per cent of diagnosed cases reported in Finland (Panchaud et al., 2000), reported incidence of syphilis (1.8 per 100,000 aged 16–19) and gonorrhoea (3.7 per 100,000 aged 16–19) are both low. The reported incidence of chlamydia is noted to be high (650.8 per 100,000 aged 16–19) (Panchaud et al., 2000); however, this may be the result of a combination of higher testing rates for chlamydia and/or higher use of oral contraceptives by young women rather than a reliance on condoms.

Fewer young people in Finland use condoms than in the Netherlands, either as a single or combined method. This may have occurred as a result of the lack of availability of condoms in Finland until the late 1980s (Väestöliitto, 1994), coupled with the lack of concern among young people in Finland about the threat of HIV, resulting from the fact that the number of cases until the end of the 1998 was very low (EuroHIV, 2000). In recent years, however, increasing incidence of HIV has raised awareness of the need to promote both condoms and oral contraceptives (Hosie, 2001) and national sexual health surveys of young people have begun to explore the use, and in turn promote the practice, of 'Double-Dutch' contraceptive methods (Liinamo, 2000).

By the mid-1990s Finland had witnessed a dramatic decline in abortion rates to young women under 20 and key organizations suggested that a level of complacency about the successful reduction in this negative outcome had set in among government and local level institutions, including schools (Hosie, 2001). Since 1995 the pregnancy rate to young women aged 15–19 in Finland has risen slowly but notably, and practitioners and researchers in Finland have suggested that this has occurred as a result of the cutbacks noted above (Hosie, 2001; STAKES, 2000: personal communication in Hosie, 2001; Kosunen, 2000; Liinamo, 2000).

Figure 4.6 outlines the trends in live birth to young women aged 15–19 from 1966–99 and abortion rates from 1980–99. An almost continual decline in both abortion and birth rates occurred until the mid-1990s; after this, the overall pregnancy rate rose for five consecutive years after 1995 (with a significant rise in abortion). Whilst the rate of reported first intercourse by 16 has increased, average levels of sexual knowledge and condom usage have both decreased (Kosunen *et al.*, 2000; Hosie, 2002).

Conclusion

With an acute awareness of the cultural context within which policy is developed and the potential impact it can have on the effectiveness of policy

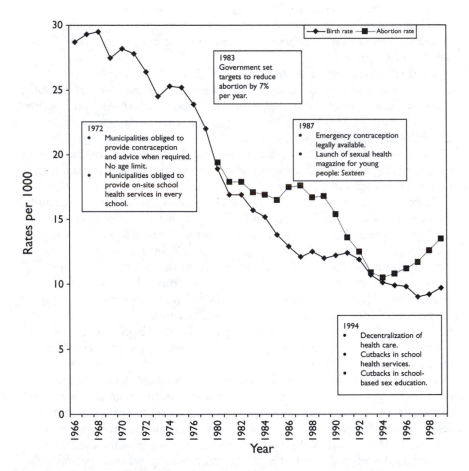

Figure 4.6 Finnish birth rates per 1000 women aged 15–19, 1966–99; abortion rates per 1000 women aged 15–19, 1980–99

Sources: Gissler, 1999; Hosie, 2001

approaches, there is nevertheless a great deal that can be learnt from exploring policy development and implementation across countries, in terms of choices about what to do as well as what not to do (Madison, 1980).

Exploring the approach to teenage sexual health promotion in Finland and the Netherlands throws light on how these countries may have achieved relative success (and in Finland's case the beginning of the reversal of that success) in reducing some of the negatives outcomes of teenage sexual behaviour over the last three decades. It helps us to understand the potential role that social policy has played in this success and highlights lessons for other countries.

Finland and the Netherlands offer similar 'success' stories in relation to the sexual health promotion of young people. The Finnish system up until 1994 offered a combination of school health services, liberal sex education provided in mixed teaching environments and an educational ethos encouraging further education; the Dutch system has youth clinics, liberal sex education and an education system that structurally encourages young people to remain at school.

However, Finland acts as a warning over complacency. Following three decades of successful promotion of young people sexual health, two recent policy changes affecting school health service provision and sex education appear to have undone 25 years of 'good practice', as evidenced by rising rates of teenage pregnancy.

In exploring case studies such as these it is important to look at combinations of policies, since no single policy is independent of others. It is also important to recognize the cultural and social factors that help to create and facilitate the acceptance of social policy, and how these will inevitably influence the extent to which policy approaches from one country may be successfully applied to any other country. However, the two countries explored here show that even cultural contexts can shift. For example, both the Netherlands and Finland have gone through a process of great change in their social attitudes towards sexual health and this has been accompanied by significant advances in the promotion of young people's sexual health. This provides lessons for more conservative countries, where policy makers often use less liberal social attitudes as reasons not to develop policy in sensitive areas when there might in fact be an equally valid case for using policy as a way of helping to shift broader social attitudes.

References

Age of Consent Finland: http://www.ageofconsent.com/finland.htm accessed 17/03/2003.

Age of Consent Netherlands: http://www.ageofconsent.com/netherlands. htm accessed 17/03/2003.

Aggleton, P., Oliver, C. and Rivers, K. (1999) *The Implications of Research into Young People, Sex, Sexuality and Relationships*. London: Health Education Authority.

Allen, I. (1991) *Family Planning and Pregnancy Counselling Projects for Young People*. London: Policy Studies Institute.

Beets, G. (1999a) Education and age at first birth. *DEMOS*, August: special edition.

Beets, G. (1999b) NIDI project 100.01: Fertility and family surveys. *DEMOS*, August: Special edition.

Bloxham, S., Capstick, S. and Greenwood, A. (1999) Combining GUM and contraceptive services for young people: profile of an innovative clinic, *British Journal of Family Planning*, **25**: 18–21.

de Bruijn, E. and Howieson, C. (1995) Modular vocational education and training in Scotland and the Netherlands: between specificity and coherence. *Comparative Education* 31(1): 83–99.

Cheesbrough, S., Ingham, R. and Massey, D. (1999) *Reducing the Rate of Teenage Conceptions – An International Review of the Evidence: USA, Canada, Australia and New Zealand*. London: HEA.

Clements, S. *et al.* (1997) *Modelling the Spatial Distribution of Teenage Conception Rates within Wessex*. University of Southampton: Centre for Sexual Health Research.

David, H. P. (1992) Abortion in Europe, 1920–1991: a public health perspective. *Studies of Family Planning* 23: 1–22.

Davis, S. (1989) Pregnancy in adolescents. *Paediatric Clinic North America* **36**: 665–80.

DfES (2002) *Public Service Agreement*, www.dfes.gov.uk/psa2002/

EC/Eurydice/Eurostat (2000) *Key data on education in Europe: Chapter E: Secondary education*. European Commission.

EuroHIV (2000) *HIV/AIDS Surveillance in Europe: Mid-Year Report 2000* 63. France: EuroHIV/UNAIDS/ WHO.

Family Planning Association (1994) *Young People's Attitudes Towards Sex Education*. London: FPA.

Francis, C. (1984) Sex education for teenagers in Holland. *Nursing Standard* 8(15): 27–31.

Fullerton, D., Dickson, R. and Sheldon, T. (1997) Preventing and reducing the adverse effects of teenage pregnancy. *Health Visitor* 70(5): 197–9.

Gissler, M. (ed.) (1999) Aborter i Norden-Induced Abortions in the Nordic Countries, *Tilastoraportti-Statistical Report* 10, Helsinki.

Hadley, A. (1998) *Getting Real: Improving Teenage Sexual Health*. Fabian Society, London: College Hill Press.

Hofmann, A. D. (1984) Contraception in adolescence: a review, 1. Psychosocial aspects, *Bulletin WHO* 62: 161–2.

Hosie, A. (2001) *A Comparative Exploration of Social Policy Relating to Teenage Pregnancy in Finland and Scotland*. Unpublished doctoral thesis, Stirling University.

Hosie, A. (2002) *Evidence into Action: Sexual Health Policy Analysis in Selected European Countries*, Edinburgh: HEBS.

Hosie, A. and Silver, C. (2001) Overcoming the first hurdle – young people and access to sexual health services in Scotland, England, Finland and the Netherlands. *European Population Conference*, Helsinki, 7–9 June 2001.

ISD Scotland (2000a) *Genitourinary Medicine Statistics Scotland*. Edinburgh: ISD Scotland.

ISD Scotland (2000b) Teenage pregnancy in Scotland 1990–2000. *Health Briefing* **99**(4), June 2000.

Jones, E. F., Forrest, J. D., Goldman, N., Henshaw, S. K., Lincoln, R., Rosoff, J. I., Westoff, C. F. and Wulf, D. (1985) Teenage pregnancy in developed countries: determinants and policy implications. *Family Planning Perspectives* **17**: 53–63.

Jones, E. F., Forrest, J. D., Goldman, N., Henshaw, S. K., Lincoln, R., Rosoff, J. I., Westoff, C. and Wulf, D. (1986) *Teenage Pregnancy in Industrialized Countries.* New Haven and London: Yale University Press.

Kane, R. and Wellings, K. (1999) *Reducing the Rate of Teenage Conceptions – An International Review of the Evidence: Data from Europe.* London: HEA.

Ketting, E. and Schnabel, P. (1980) Induced abortion in the Netherlands: a decade of experience, 1970–1980. *Studies in Family Planning* **11**(12): 385–94.

Kontula, O. and Rimpelä, M. (1988) The knowledge of young people on sexual development, in L. Kannas and S. Miilunpalo (eds), *Terveyskasvatus- tustkimusken vuosikirja, Lääkintöhalliyuksen julkaisuja. Terveyskasvatus.* Sarja Tutkimukset 8. Tampere.

Kosunen, E. (1993) *Teini-ikäisten rasaudet ja ehkäisy.* Vol. 99, Jyväskylä: Gummerus Kirjapaino, STAKES.

Kosunen, E. (1996) *Adolescent Reproductive Health in Finland: Oral Contraception, Pregnancies and Abortions from the 1980s to the 1990s.* Tampere: doctoral thesis, *Acta Universitatis Tamperensis* ser A Vol.486.

Kosunen, E. (2000) Adolescent sexual health, in I. Lottes and O. Kontula, *New Views on Sexual Health: The Case of Finland.* Series D 37/2000. Helsinki: Population Research Institute.

Kosunen, E. and Rimpelä, M. (1996) Improving adolescence sexual health in Finland. *Choices: Sexual Health and Family Planning in Europe* **25**: 18–21.

Kosunen, E., Rimpelä, M., Liinamo, A. and Jokela, J. (2000) Sumalaistenn- uorten seksuaalikäyttäytymisen muutpkset 1990-luvun lopulla. *Journal of Social Medicine* **37**: 273–82.

Liinamo, A. (2000) Sex education in Finland, in I. Lottes and O. Kontula, *New Views on Sexual Health: The Case of Finland.* Series D 37. Helsinki: Population Research Institute.

Liinamo, A. *et al.* (1997) Taking adolescents seriously: four areas of Finland, in A. Hardon and E. Hayes, *Reproductive Rights in Practice: A Feminist Report on the Quality of Care.* London: Zed.

Madison, B. (1980) *The Meaning of Social Policy: The Comparative Dimension in Social Welfare.* London: Croom Helm.

McIlwaine, G. (1994) *Needs Assessment: A National Approach – Teenage Pregnancy in Scotland.* Glasgow: SNAP (Scottish Needs Assessment Programme), Scottish Forum for Public Health Medicine.

Morrison, D. M. (1985) Adolescent contraception behaviour: a review. *Psychological Bulletin* **98**(3): 538–68.

National Board of Education (1998) *The Scholastic Programs of Sexual Education in Finland.* Helsinki: NBE.

Nelson, F. (1997) Why is gender a barrier to contraception advice? *Nursing Times* **93**(6): 50–2.

NHS Centre for Reviews and Dissemination (1997) Prevention and reducing the adverse effects of unintended teenage pregnancies. *Effective Healthcare Bulletin* **3**(1).

Panchaud, C., Singh, S., Feivelson, D. and Darroch, J. E. (2000) Sexually transmitted diseases among adolescents in developed countries. *Family Planning Perspectives* **32**(1): 24–32, 45.

Papp, K. (1997) Knowledge of sexual issues, moral beliefs, and sexual experiences among adolescence in Estonia and Finland. *Research Reports* **82**. Jyväskylä: STAKES.

Peckham, S. (1993) Preventing unintended teenage pregnancies. *Public Health* **107**: 123–33.

Pryor, M. (2001) *Abortion in the Netherlands*. http://www.lifeissues.net/writers/pry/index.html

Rademakers, J. (1991) *Interactie en Anticonceptie: De Preventie van Ongewenste Zwangerschap Door Jongeren in Nederland*. Den Haag: Cip-Gegevens Koninklijke Bibliotheek.

Röling, H. (1993) Sexual knowledge as the boundary between youth and adulthood and the ideal of sexual innocence in the Dutch debate on sexual instruction 1890–1960. *Paedagogica Historica* **29**: 229–40.

Ross, J. and Wyatt, W. (2000) Sexual behaviour, in C. Currie, K. Hurrelmann, W. Settertobulte, R. Smith and J. Todd, *Health Behaviour in School-Aged Children: A WHO Cross-National Study (HBSC) International Report*. Denmark: World Health Organization Regional Office for Europe.

Selman, P. and Glendinning, C. (1996) Teenage pregnancy: do social policies make a difference? in J. Brannen and M. O'Brien, *Children and Families: Research and Social Policy*. London: Falmer.

Sheldon, T. (1997) The Dutch experience. *Heathlines*, April: 12–13.

Sheldon, T. (1998) Sex in the classroom – Dutch style. *Heathlines*, Dec 97–Jan 98.

Silver, C. (1998) *Prevent or Accept?: A Qualitative Comparison of the Content, Provision and Effectiveness of Sex Education in England and Wales and the Netherlands*. Unpublished M.Sc. dissertation, University of Surrey, Guildford.

Silver, C. (1999) *Dutch Society – In Historical Context*. Unpublished paper. University of Surrey, Guildford.

Singh, S. and Darroch, J.E. (2000) Adolescent pregnancy and childbearing: levels and trends in developed countries. *Family Planning Perspectives* **32**(1): 14–23.

Social Exclusion Unit (1999) *Teenage Pregnancy*. London: The Stationery Office.

Thompson, J. (1976) Fertility and abortion inside and outside marriage. *Population Trends* **5**: 3–8.

Turner, K. M. (2001) *Predictable Pathways? An Exploration of Young Women's Perceptions of Teenage Pregnancy and Early Motherhood*. Unpublished doctoral thesis, University of Stirling.

United Nations (1977) *UN Demographic Yearbooks 1976*. New York: United Nations.

United Nations (1984) *UN Demographic Yearbooks 1983*. New York: United Nations.

United Nations (1988) *Adolescence Reproductive Behaviour. Evidence from Developed Countries Vol.1*. New York: United Nations.

United Nations (1990) *UN Demographic Yearbooks 1989*. New York: United Nations.

United Nations (1997) *UN Demographic Yearbooks 1996*. New York: United Nations.

Väestöliittö (1994) *The Evolution of Reproductive Health Care in Finland: How We Did It*. Helsinki: Väestöliittö.

Vilar, D. (1994) School sex education: still a priority in Europe. *Planned Parenthood in Europe* **23**(3): 812.

Wellings, K., Field, J., Johnson, A. M. and Wadsworth, J. (1994) *Sexual Behaviour in Britain. The National Survey of Sexual Attitudes and Lifestyles*. London: Penguin.

World Bank (2001) *2.17 Reproductive Health*. www.worldbank.org/data/wdi2001/pdfs/tab2_17.pdf.

Yarrow, A. (1978) Extra-marital pregnancy in young women. *Journal of Maternal and Child Health*. May: 178–9.

Zabin, L. S., Hirsch, M. B., Smith, E. A. *et al.* (1986) Evaluation of a pregnancy prevention programme for urban teenagers. *Family Planning Perspectives* **18**(3): 119–26.

5 Sexual Health Policies and Trends in the USA, New Zealand and Australia

ROGER INGHAM
and RACHEL PARTRIDGE

> **Key issues**
>
> • Potentially valuable lessons can be learnt by comparing policies across countries however the methodological difficulties should not be underestimated.
> • National and sub-national policies undoubtedly influence the climate surrounding sexuality among young people. A more liberal climate can be protective and comprehensive interventions do not lead apparently to increased sexual activity.
> • Policy is shaped by many factors including public opinion. Advocacy, based on evidence as well as a rights perspective, can help to change policy to be more supportive of young people's sexuality.

Overview

This chapter looks at national policy developments in the USA, New Zealand and Australia and attempts to relate these to young people's sexual health outcomes. It summarizes the key patterns in each country before highlighting what the implications might be for other countries in the development of policy initiatives.

Introduction

This chapter presents sexual health data from Australia, New Zealand and the USA, including rates of teenage conceptions, abortions and sexually transmitted infections (STIs). These countries were selected since they are well developed economically, have good educational and health services infrastructures, and use English as their main language.

The chapter considers policy developments in the three countries, exploring the links that may exist with sexual health outcomes and seeking to highlight general lessons. In doing so, it is important to reiterate the provisos raised in the section overview, relating to problems with data reliability, comparability and policy tracking, and making causal links. The nature of government in the USA and Australia poses an additional difficulty, as these countries are divided into reasonably autonomous states where different laws and policies apply.

Chapter 4 shows the teenage birth and abortion rates for a number of European countries, while this chapter compares data for the USA, New Zealand and Australia. The high rates in the USA are probably the most oft-quoted statistic in sexual health research. Less frequently cited is that New Zealand's total conception rate is higher than rates in west European countries (amongst which the UK is the highest), with Australia close to the upper end of the range in west Europe. Of particular note is the higher rate of abortion in Australia.

There have been some changes in teenage birth rates in the countries over the past 20 years, as shown in Figure 5.1. While the UK and Australia were similar in 1980, the latter shows a marked reduction between 1980 and 2000. The rates in the USA and the UK have remained fairly constant during this period, whereas New Zealand has experienced a gradual decline in rates from around 38/1000 in 1980 to 29/1000, which is lower than the UK rate in 2000.

The United States of America

The USA (population 280 million) has a diverse and complex ethnic composition. Health care is delivered through private providers, with the majority

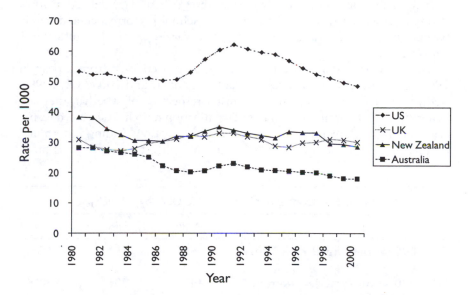

Figure 5.1 Birth rates per 1000 women aged 15–19 years, 1980–2000 (or latest available date)

of the population being covered by insurance. Some public hospitals and services are provided for the poorest sectors through Medicaid, a joint federal–state programme.

The culture regarding sexuality is very mixed. At one extreme, some areas have a reputation for liberal attitudes and tolerance. At the other extreme, there are powerful moralistic movements, with strong negative attitudes towards abortion, and negative views towards the provision of sex education and contraception services for young people. Laws and policies are developed at either federal or state level; the federal law may grant rights but states can impose their own restrictions. For example, the 'federal' age of consent for sexual intercourse is 16 years, although this varies from 12 years in Delaware to 18 years in 13 states. Similarly, within each state there are counties and districts, again with some autonomy over laws and policies.

Sexual health indices

The higher conception and birth rates in the USA apply across the teenage category; there were around 30 births per 1000 amongst 15 to 17 year olds, and 82 per 1000 amongst 18 and 19 year olds. These overall data hide quite substantial ethnic and geographic variations, as shown in Table 5.1. Although levels of sexual activity during teenage years are somewhat higher amongst the non-white populations, these differences are nowhere near large enough to account for the different conception rates. Ventura *et al.* (2000) have estimated conception rates among just those who have ever had intercourse; these are also shown in Table 5.1.

It must be borne in mind when considering these data that ethnicity is strongly associated with social deprivation, school performance and family background characteristics. There are also large geographic differences between states.

The USA has shown a decline in teenage conceptions, from a peak in 1990 of around 116 to the latest available rate of around 100 (AGI, 1999). Reductions have occurred in all states, irrespective of whether they are generally high or low in overall rates. The abortion ratio has decreased (especially amongst whites) from 46 per cent of conceptions ending in termination in 1986 to 32 per cent in 1996, indicating that a higher proportion of

Table 5.1 Conception rates in the USA, by ethnicity

	White	Hispanic	Black
Per 1000 women aged 15–19 years	68	157	178
Per 1000 sexually active women aged 15–19 years	142	291	305

Source: Ventura *et al.*, 2000

pregnant teenagers are completing their pregnancies. It is not clear whether this indicates an increase in the 'wantedness' of children, greater difficulties in obtaining abortions, or a mix of both.

There are shortcomings in the reliability of data on STIs in the USA due to the prevalence of private medical care. However, Darroch *et al.* (2001) cite Panchaud *et al.*'s work, which reports that the USA has higher rates than most other countries, with chlamydia being twice the rate of Canada and Sweden, five times the rate in England and 20 times that in France. Collins *et al.* (2002) report that one in four sexually active individuals will have had an STI by the age of 24 years.

The policy context

Sexual health services for young people are provided in a number of ways (AGI, 2000a, 2000b). The key ones include private insurance, Medicaid (which has included family planning services since 1972; in 1994 it accounted for 46 per cent of public funding of contraceptive services) and Title X (which has supported family planning and sexual health services for poorer women and young people since 1970; in 1994 it accounted for 21 per cent of public spending on family planning). These federal funding schemes have had (and still have) a chequered reception and have been repeatedly subject to strong moral and religious objections. During the conservative Reagan administration, federal funding to Title X was severely cut, and despite increases during the 1990s, it is nearly 60 per cent below what it was in 1980 (Gold, 2001). These cuts have occurred at a time of increasing pressures on services, including increasing numbers of uninsured women, increasing costs of contraceptives, greater popularity of long lasting (and more expensive) methods, and a greater diversity of needs within communities. The funding of these family planning and sexual health services – especially for young people – remains controversial and contested.

Similarly, sex education policy in the USA has a mixed history, with a series of controversial policies being introduced in recent years. Federal law does not actually require sexuality education in schools, but Congress sometimes provides funding for it. In 1981, the AFLA (Adolescent Family Life Act/'Chastity Act') was passed, designed to 'promote self discipline and other prudent approaches to the problem of adolescent premarital sexual relations, including adolescent pregnancy'. The programme awards grants to public and non-profit organizations to provide services to prevent 'premarital sexual relations and adolescent pregnancy', as well as supporting pregnant young people and teenage parents.

The 1996 welfare reform legislation contained a more restrictive eight-point definition of abstinence education, including tenets such as:

- Abstinence from sexual activity is the only certain way to avoid out-of-wedlock pregnancy, STIs, and other associated health problems.

- Sexual activity outside of the context of marriage is likely to have harmful psychological and physical effects.
- Bearing children out of wedlock is likely to have harmful consequences for the child, the child's parents, and society.

This abstinence-only policy is popular with the G. W. Bush administration, and the programme has received $135 million of federal funding. This marks a 3000 per cent rise in funding between 1996 and 2001 (Advocates for Youth, 2001).

A survey by the Alan Guttmacher Institute (AGI) showed that 86 per cent of school districts with a sexuality education policy require the promotion of abstinence, with either no coverage of contraception or coverage limited to information on failure rates. Hence only 14 per cent of schools have 'truly comprehensive' policies, despite evidence that the vast majority of teachers, parents and young people prefer more comprehensive coverage (Dailard, 2001).

Despite the wide coverage and strong financing for abstinence-only education, there is little evidence that the approach is more successful than a more holistic, integrated approach to sexual health education. In a series of comprehensive evaluations of school-based programmes, Kirby (2001) highlights the lack of rigorous evaluation of abstinence-only programs, in contrast to a large body of evaluation research showing that:

> sex and HIV education programs do not increase sexual activity – they do not hasten the onset of sex, increase the frequency of sex, nor increase the number of sexual partners. To the contrary, some ... delay the onset of sex, reduce the frequency of sex or reduce the number of partners.

Other research has suggested that abstinence programmes may lead to a slight delay in first intercourse. However, there is a decreased use of contraception when sex does occur, and greater pressure on those young women who do not follow the abstinence advice (those who do not sign 'the pledge') (Bearman and Brueckner, 1998).

Singh and Darroch (1999) conclude that around one-quarter of the decline in sexual activity and conception rates can be attributed to the growth of abstinence programmes, with the remaining three-quarters of the decline being credited to increased information and services regarding contraception.

In conclusion, although there are clear variations between ethnic groups in terms of teenage pregnancy and birth rates, the levels amongst white Americans are still higher than for other developed countries. The difficulties involved in getting reliable information on precisely when different policies were introduced at state and more local levels render the task of making direct links between policy changes and sexual health outcomes virtually impossible.

Whatever political party is in power, there has been a strong ideological and financial encouragement for morality and abstinence education, although the available data do not suggest that this is a major factor in accounting for the recent decline in teenage pregnancy rates.

New Zealand

New Zealand (population 3.8 million) has a mixed population, with 10 per cent identifying as Maori in the 1966 census, and a further 4 per cent as Asian (mainly Pacific Islanders). The remainder of the population is of European descent, known as Päkehä, or NZ Europeans. The general view of sexuality in recent years can be described as 'conservative' and this appears to have affected the provision of services for young people, the level of school-based education, and general cultural attitudes.

Sexual health indices

Total conception rates for New Zealand teenagers were estimated at around 65 per thousand women aged between 15 and 19 in 1997 (Dickson *et al.*, 2000). There is a relatively high rate of teenage births, at around 29 per thousand in 2000, and there are large differences between ethnic groups (Figure 5.2).

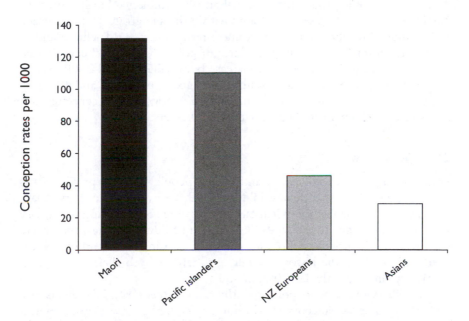

Figure 5.2 Estimated conception rates per 1000 women aged 15–19 years, by ethnicity

Source: Dickson *et al.*, 2000

The birth rate among the Maori teenagers has been consistently around 2 to 2.5 times higher than among NZ European teenagers, and has been rising over the past few years. The difference reflects in part the link between ethnicity and social deprivation (and the latter's link with teenage mother-hood), and also different cultural attitudes towards early marriage and child-bearing. Since the non-European population represents around 15 per cent of the total population, and using the 1995 data, the rate amongst the NZ European population can be roughly estimated as being around 29, still higher than Australia and Canada, similar to the UK and around half of the US rate.

The latest available data on abortions (Statistics New Zealand, 2001) give a figure of 23.5 per thousand for the 15 to 19 age group. Dickson *et al.* (2000) estimate the proportions of conceptions ending in abortion at 24 per cent among Maori, 72 per cent among Asians, and 54 per cent among NZ Europeans. The proportions of overall teenage conceptions that have been terminated have increased from 31 per cent in 1983, to 37 per cent in 1995, to 40 per cent in 1997 (Dickson *et al.*, 2000). Among all groups, the proportions of teenage births that occurred within marriage reduced from 54 per cent in 1976 to 5 per cent in 1994–5.

STI rates are increasing, although data are limited. (Dickson *et al.*, 1996; Lyttle and Preston, 1997) Confirmed cases of chlamydia increased by 23 per cent between 1999 and 2000. The increase is reported as occurring in all age, sex and ethnic groups (draft Sexual and Reproductive Health Strategy, 2001); 34 per cent of cases were found within the age group 15 to 19 years, and considerably higher rates were found among Maori and Pacific Islanders than other ethnic groups. Similarly, rates of gonorrhoea have been increasing since 1996, with a 28 per cent increase between 1999 and 2000. Again, 37 per cent of cases occurred among those aged between 15 and 19 years. Fifty per cent of all cases were found among Maori, 28 per cent amongst European and 16 per cent amongst Pacific Islanders.

The policy context

Policy relating to sex education and young people's service provision has been a topic of intense debate in New Zealand over recent years. Clark (2001) outlines the history of legislation regarding sex education in primary schools, beginning with the 1945 Department of Education view that 'there is no place in the primary school for group or class instruction in sex educa-tion' and labelling the history overall as a 'tangled web skein of morality, religion, politics and the law' (pp. 23–30).

The 1954 Government-sponsored *Mazengarb Report* had 27 conclusions, one stating that 'adolescents should not buy or be in possession of contra-ceptives', in response to which a law was passed making it illegal to supply contraceptives to young people under 16; providing instruction or persua-sion regarding contraceptive use were also made illegal (Sparrow, 1991).

This meant that, legally, no one – neither teachers nor parents – could let under-16s know about contraception.

This situation characterized New Zealand's approach to young people's sexuality until the 1977 Contraception, Sterilisation and Abortion (CSA) Bill was passed. This covered three areas: it enabled authorized persons to provide contraceptives to those under 16 years, to direct or persuade an under 16 year old to use any contraception, and instruct an under 16 year old in the use of any contraceptive. However, whilst the situation for 'authorized persons' (that is, doctors) was clarified, the situation for many others was uncertain, media coverage of contraception was still restricted, and condom vending machines could not be placed where under-16s might have access. This section of the CSA act was not repealed until 1990, in the face of mounting pressure from human rights lobby groups and the advent of HIV/AIDS.

More recently, a new health education syllabus was introduced with clear provision for sex education in primary schools, and a distinction has been made between 'sex' education and 'sexuality' education. A recent internal policy paper produced by a Government department as a contribution towards the new Sexual Health Strategy reports that:

> In 1996 the Education Review Office reported that sexuality education was often poor and piecemeal. Many schools were not delivering programmes in accordance with the national curriculum statement and some young people were not receiving any sexuality education.

The report refers to the new curriculum, mentioned above, but adds that while it was due to be implemented in all schools by the beginning of 2001 it has not yet been mandated and so is not yet compulsory (NZ Ministry of Youth Affairs, 2001).

Abortion has also had a particularly controversial position in New Zealand legislation and there has been no change in the 1977 CSA law which relates to the provision of abortion. The Abortion Supervisory Committee (ASC) (established in 1977 to oversee the operation of the CSA Act), as well as other public welfare lobby groups, have been frustrated at the general lack of Government action:

> If abortion is abhorrent to the majority of our thinking population, then the emphasis should be on education aimed at achieving a higher proportion of planned pregnancies than perpetuating the present unwieldy system of authorising the termination of potentially normal pregnancies on pseudo-legal grounds.
>
> (ASC, 1988: 3)

> The [CSA] Act is outdated in its language and content. Its procedures are too complex and are not being followed as the law intended. Its provisions for providing legal, safe abortions are not being consistently applied

throughout the country. The act is demeaning to women in requiring a medical procedure to be considered under the Crimes Act. It is also misleading that 98.2 per cent of abortions have to be granted under mental health provisions.

(ASC, 2000: 5)

Recently, however, there have been signs of change in New Zealand. A draft Sexual Health Strategy was prepared in 2001 by the Minister of Health, acknowledging the need to involve other sectors including education, families and communities, and paying special attention to the Maori population. The Strategy was produced in consultation with a reference group, which included academic researchers, clinicians, schools, family planning organizations and sex workers. Four strategic directions are identified – societal attitudes, values and behaviour; personal knowledge, skills and behaviour; services; information – and action plans are anticipated for specific issues.

In conclusion, sexual health policies in New Zealand appear to have been characterized by opposition and conflict. Rates of teenage conceptions were relatively high in the mid-1970s, with over half occurring within marriage. However, since this time, and whilst the government has been prevaricating about the laws, the conception rate amongst teenagers has not been declining. The proportions of these conceptions that led to births have, however, been decreasing over the past 20 years. Despite the clear difficulties in obtaining terminations, the numbers carried out have increased markedly. This picture suggests that insufficient attention has been paid to prevention, and that the recently produced sexual health strategy is timely.

There are large variations between ethnic groups in the country, with Maori and Pacific Islanders having considerably higher rates of teenage conceptions than the NZ Europeans. The relative contributions of cultural heritage and economic deprivation to these patterns are not easy to disentangle.

Australia

Australia (population 19 million) has a mixed population, 2 to 3 per cent indigenous (Aboriginal and Torres Strait Islanders), a growing Asian population, and many from diverse European origins. There are seven states/territories, each with powers to enact laws and policies within the framework of the national government (known as 'the Commonwealth').

In relation to sexual health, Australia is often regarded as being fairly liberal. The response to the threat of HIV and AIDS was comparatively rapid, and there are a number of long-standing dedicated research centres based in universities.

Sexual health indices

Australia has the lowest teenage birth rate of the countries considered here (18.4 per 1000 in 1998), with substantial regional and ethnic variation.

While Aboriginal and Torres Strait Islander communities are only a small proportion of the total population, the birth rate to teenage indigenous aboriginal women is high with around 27 per cent of all births occurring to women under 20 compared to 6 per cent among non-indigenous women (Siedlecky, 1996). The Northern Territory has the highest teenage rate at 67.6 births per 1000 females aged 15–19 years (Australian Bureau of Statistics, 2000). Although national data on terminations are not yet available, data from the state of South Australia and from the Northern Territory (both of which have specific abortion legislation) show an abortion ratio among teenagers in 1996 of around 50 per cent (Moon et al., 1999).

Australia is the only one of the three countries to show a consistent decline in teenage births over the past 30 years. A birth rate that was comparable to the UK in the 1970s and early 1980s has fallen markedly to the lowest ever rate of 18.1 births per 1000 15 to 19 year old women in 1999 (Australian Bureau of Statistics, 2000).

STI surveillance data indicate that sexually active young people in the 13–19 age group are at high risk; in 1996, this group constituted 23 per cent of chlamydia infections (Lindsay et al., 1997). The rate of diagnosis of chlamydia has more than doubled over the past five years (Annual Surveillance Report, 2000). Notifications of gonococcal infections amongst young people have also increased during the period 1991 to 1998, from 31 to 65 per 100,000. Indigenous people continue to be diagnosed with STIs at a much higher rate.

The policy context

The decrease in teenage birth rates since 1971 has been partly attributed to the reinterpretation of abortion laws, such as the amendment of the law in Northern Territory in 1969 and 1974 to define lawful abortion (UN, 1992), and to a greater willingness of medical practitioners to prescribe contraceptives, particularly the contraceptive pill, to unmarried women (Moon et al., 1999). It could also be influenced by a cultural shift towards safer sexual practices, such as increased condom use, which has been stimulated by increased discussion about sexual health issues and by school-based sex education classes since the emergence of HIV in Australia in 1982.

The Australian government responded comparatively quickly to the advent of HIV/AIDS. Policy statements and teachers' guides have been circulated through secondary schools since the mid-1980s with suggestions for sex education for students including STIs, HIV and modes of transmission, safer sex and homosexuality (Goldman and Goldman, 1992). Although states and territories vary in curriculum guidelines and mandated time spent on health education, they all place sexuality and drug education within the learning area of Health and Physical Education (ANCHARD, 1999). More recently, in response to results from a survey revealing continuing fairly high levels of unsafe sex amongst young people, the Commonwealth Department of Health and Family Services hosted a meeting of state and territory government and non-government representatives in 1998. This helped to develop a national framework for education about STIs, HIV/AIDS, and blood borne viruses in schools. The output from this event led to a resource that helps in developing educational programmes in schools (ANCHARD, 1999).

In the absence of a national sexual health strategy, policy direction for Australia's response to sexual health issues has come from a variety of areas. At the national level, the National HIV/AIDS strategy 1996–7 to 1998–9 is described in its title as being 'framed within the context of sexual health'. The strategy calls for a coordinated approach to policy development to deal with HIV and other STIs, and that the clinical approach to STI prevention and management should be complemented with programs of peer education and community development (McCallum *et al.*, 2000).

Several other documents have also provided strategic direction for the development of HIV/AIDS and sexual health services and programmes, including the Australian Federation of AIDS Organizations (AFAO) discussion papers and the National Indigenous Australians' Sexual Health Strategy 1995–6 to 1998–9.

National strategic direction is also provided in the non-government sector: for example, the work of the family planning programme agencies and a significant component of Commonwealth funding to family planning organizations (FPOs) has been for clinical training for health professionals.

All state and territory capital cities in Australia have a sexual health service or clinic, either as a sexual health centre or as an outpatient clinic attached to a public hospital. The National HIV/AIDS Strategy provided states and territories with the flexibility to channel Commonwealth AIDS funds into the development or expansion of sexual health services. In recent years, there has been an expansion of services from family planning or HIV/AIDS focused services to include sexual health and other communicable diseases, which, in turn, has meant an increase in accessible services for young people. Many state and territory family planning organizations have established regional clinics and have some outreach services, whilst also providing specific clinical and health promotion services for young people; for example, the SHine programme in South Australia, has adopted a decentralized and explicit primary health care model for the provision of a broad range of prevention, health education and clinical sexual health services.

Furthermore, in response to the results of a national survey of school children in Years 10 and 12 which revealed that general practitioners and local doctors were particularly important sources of advice on HIV, STIs and contraception (Lindsay *et al.*, 1997), the National Divisions Youth Alliance made a submission before the Commonwealth aimed at coordinating the work of divisions of general practice in relation to youth services, with sexual health as a priority area (McCallum *et al.*, 2000).

However, there are still some areas relating to sexual health that are not well covered, with reform being slow and complicated by the differing state and territory legislation; these include illegal immigrant sex workers, the age of consent and termination of pregnancy.

In conclusion, Australia appears to have adopted a pragmatic approach to the sexual health threats facing young people, and their rates have shown a steady decline over the past 30 years. Despite the absence of a formal sexual health strategy, changes appear to have occurred within the education and service sectors in relation to sexual health. Although there are undoubtedly opposing voices to increasing provision, these have not had the impact on policies and progress in the way characterized by New Zealand and the USA.

Conclusion

This chapter indicates a wide range of policy positions, sexual health patterns and cultural attitudes across these three relatively rich countries. It has shown tremendous variation at any given time within countries, especially in the cases of the USA and Australia with their complex political systems. The factors that underlie these variations are less clear and differences in data types and time points militate against making hard and fast comparisons.

With just three countries, direct correlations between sexual health indices and other aspects of societies are simply not feasible; much larger samples are required to attempt this. For example, employment rates amongst young people, the proportions of young people remaining in full-time education, income distribution patterns, patterns of welfare payments, and so on, have all been suggested as factors that affect teenage conception rates. However, of the three countries considered here, Australia has the highest youth unemployment rate and the lowest average years' schooling amongst women, and yet has the lowest teenage conception rates.

General cultural attitudes and norms towards young people's sexuality appear to be crucial. However, in the absence of periodic national surveys that directly assess such norms, these can only be inferred.

Despite these difficulties, and the problems of attributing change to specific changes in policies and laws, some general conclusions can be drawn, especially when considered alongside the results of other reviews that have considered a wider range of countries and indices, including those conducted by Cheesbrough *et al.* (1999), Kane and Wellings (1999) UNICEF (2001), Hosie (see Chapter 4) and Darroch *et al.* (2001).

- A more liberal climate towards sexuality among young people appears to be protective. The USA and New Zealand have been characterized by intense disputes over the way forward – with accompanying prevarications and delays – and have higher rates of teenage pregnancy. Australia, conversely, is regarded as being more liberal and has lower rates of teenage conceptions. The Alan Guttmacher Institute analysis in the USA supports this conclusion, and attributes the majority of the recent reduction in rates to improved contraception provision, rather than to the efforts of the abstinence movement.

- Comparative reviews of five developed countries (Singh *et al.*, 2001; Darroch *et al.*, 2001) point to two major factors that help to account for the large national differences:
  - o The extent of socioeconomic disadvantage is considerably higher in the USA than in its comparator countries (Canada, Sweden, France and Great Britain), and it accounts for much of the variation between rates of teenage conception rates in the countries.
  - o Differences in the numbers of young people who are sexually active at comparable ages are insufficient to account for the variations in rates. Rather, they point to the regularity of contraceptive use as the major factor. This implies that efforts to reduce the onset of sexual activity are less likely to have a large impact than efforts to improve availability and use of contraception.
- It is difficult to directly attribute change to specific activities. Comprehensive reviews of new school programmes and other forms of intervention frequently conclude that results are mixed. However, most are confident that, at the very least, new and more open programmes do not lead to increased sexual activity. The importance of this conclusion cannot be overstated given the barriers that are apparent in the USA and New Zealand (and some other countries).

Finally, the climate surrounding sexuality among young people affects a range of areas and approaches, including the provision and style of education, service provision, the attitudes of staff within these services, the interpretation of policies, patterns of communication within and outside families, and so on. National and sub-national policies undoubtedly influence this climate and may be a mechanism for changing it, preferably based on research data rather than on dogma, political rhetoric and unfounded beliefs.

In some cases, such change may reflect and respond to changing public opinion, rather than lead to it. In other cases, confident and well-informed leadership and advocacy can be an important component of creating a climate in which young people and their sexual health concerns are more fully respected.

References

ASC (1988) *Abortion Supervisory Committee of New Zealand Annual Report 1998*, presented to the House of Representatives pursuant to Section 39 of the CSA Act 1977.

ASC (2000) *Abortion Supervisory Committee of New Zealand Annual Report 2000*, presented to the House of Representatives pursuant to Section 39 of the CSA Act 1977.

Advocates for Youth (2001) *Toward a Sexually Healthy America; Roadblocks*

Imposed by the Federal Government's Abstinence-Only-Until-Marriage Education Programme. www.advocatesforyouth.org/publications/abstinenceonly.pdf

Alan Guttmacher Institute (AGI) (1999) *Teenage Pregnancy; Overall Trends and State-By-State Information,* http://www.agi-usa.org/pubs/teen_preg_stats.html

AGI (2000a) *US Policy Can Reduce the Cost of Barriers to Contraception, Issues in Brief.* New York: AGI.

AGI (2000b) *Fulfilling the Promise; Public Policy and US Family Planning Clinics.* New York: AGI.

Annual Surveillance Report (2000) *HIV/AIDS, Hepatitis C and Sexually Transmissable Infections in Australia.* Sydney: National Centre in HIV Epidemiology and Clinical Research.

Australian Bureau of Statistics (2000) *Population Special article – Teenage Fertility. Australian Demographic Statistics,* June quarter 2000. Canberra: Australian Bureau of Statistics

Australian National Council for HIV, Hepatitis C and Related Diseases (ANCHARD) (1999) *Talking about Sexual Health: National Framework for Education about STIs, HIV/AIDS and BBVs in Secondary Schools.* Canberra: ANCHARD.

Bearman, P. and Brueckner, H. (1998) The structure of commitment: social context and the transition to first intercourse amongst American adolescents, paper presented at the *International Academy of Sex Research* 24th annual meeting, Sirmione, Italy, June.

Cheesbrough, S., Ingham, R. and Massey, D. (1999) *Reducing the Rate of Teenage Conceptions – An International Review of the Evidence: USA, Canada, Australia and New Zealand.* London: Health Education Authority.

Clark, J. (2001) Sex education in the New Zealand primary schools; a tangled web skein of morality, religion, politics and the law. *Sex Education* 1(1): 23–30.

Collins, C., Alagiri, P., Summers, T. and Morin, S. (2002) *Abstinence Only vs. Comprehensive Sex Education; What are the Arguments, What is the Evidence?* University of California, San Francisco: AIDS Research Institute.

Dailard, C. (2001) Sex education: politicians, parents, teachers and teens. *The Guttmacher Report on Public Policy,* Feb, 4(1).

Darroch, J. E., Singh, S., Frost, J. J. and the study team (2001) Differences in teenage pregnancy rates among five developed countries; the roles of sexual activity and contraceptive use. *Family Planning Perspectives* 33(6): 244–50, 281.

Dickson, N., Paul, C., Herbison, P., McNoe, B. and Silva, P. (1996) The lifetime occurrence of sexually transmitted diseases among a cohort aged 21. *New Zealand Medical Journal,* 23 Aug: 308–11.

Dickson, N., Sporle, A., Rimene, C. and Paul, C. (2000) Pregnancies among New Zealand teenagers; trends, current status and international comparisons. *New Zealand Medical Journal,* 23 Jun: 241–5.

Gold, R. B. (2001) Title X: three decades of accomplishment. *The Guttmacher Report on Public Policy.* Feb, 4(1).

Goldman, R. and Goldman, J. (1992) *An Overview of School Based HIV/AIDS Educational Programs in Australia.* University of Queensland: National Centre for HIV Social Research.

Kane, R. and Wellings, K. (1999) *Reducing the Rate of Teenage Conceptions – An International Review of the Evidence; Data From Europe*. London: Health Education Authority.

Kirby, D. (2001) Understanding what works and what doesn't in reducing adolescent sexual risk-taking. *Family Planning Perspectives* 33(6): 276–81.

Lindsay, J., Smith, A. and Rosenthal, D. (1997) *Secondary Students, HIV/AIDS and Sexual Health*. La Trobe University, Melbourne: Centre for the Study of Sexually Transmissible Diseases.

Lyttle, H. and Preston, J. (1997) Sexually transmitted diseases and activities in New Zealand STD / Sexual Health clinics 1995. *Venereology* 10(1): 43–7.

McCallum, L., McDonald, J. and Neilsen, G. (2000) *Analysis of Current National Sexual Health Related Activities, Policies and Programs Funded by the Commonwealth – A Consultation on the Appropriateness and Scope of a National Sexual Health Strategy*. September 2000, unpublished draft final report, Sydney.

Moon, L., Meyer, P. and Grau, J. (1999) *Australia's Young People: Their Health and Wellbeing*. Canberra: Australian Institute of Health and Welfare.

New Zealand Ministry of Health (2001) *Sexual and Reproductive Health Strategy* (draft). Jul, Auckland.

New Zealand Ministry of Youth Affairs (2001) *Young People's Sexual and Reproductive Health*. Internal policy paper, Aug, Auckland.

Siedlecky, S. (1996) What is happening with teenage pregnancies? *Actuarial Studies and Demography, Research Paper Series 3*. Macquarie University, Sydney.

Singh, S. and Darroch, J. (1999) *Why is Teenage Pregnancy Declining? The Roles of Abstinence, Sexual Activity and Contraceptive Use*. Occasional Report, Washington: Alan Guttmacher Institute.

Singh, S., Darroch, J. E., Frost, J.J . and the study team (2001) Socioeconomic disadvantage and adolescent women's sexual and reproductive behavior; the case of five developed countries. *Family Planning Perspectives* 33(6): 251–8, 289.

Sparrow, M. (1991) The law relating to contraception and under-16s in New Zealand, 1954–1990. *Venereology* 4(4): 120–2.

Statistics New Zealand (2001) *Demographic Trends 2000*. Wellington: Statistics NZ.

United Nations Department of Economic and Social Development (1992) *Abortion policies: a global review*. Volume I, New York: United Nations.

UNICEF (2001) A league table of teenage births in rich nations, *Innocenti Report Card No. 3*. Florence, Italy: UNICEF Innocenti Research Centre

Ventura, S. J., Mosher, W. D., Curtin, S. C., Abma, J. C. and Henshaw, S. (2000) Trends in pregnancies and pregnancy rates by outcome; estimates for the United States, 1976–96. *Vital and Health Statistics*, 21(56). National Center for Health Statistics.

Part Three

Groups Requiring Additional Support

Inequalities in health

As with many aspects of health, who you are matters in terms of the issues you are likely to face and the support you are likely to need, want, and be offered in relation to sexual health. Where you live, what your family background and economic status are, what schools you attend, who your friends are, what your sexual orientation is – all these have an influence on sexual health outcomes, in particular for young people who may need additional support.

Over the last 20 years, the public health agenda in the UK has been dominated by a focus on these inequalities, recognising the persistent, and in some cases widening, differences in health outcomes between groups (Acheson, 1998; Treasury, 2002; Scottish Executive, 2003). At the same time, the key position of children and young people with regard to health inequalities has been highlighted (Mielck *et al.*, 2001; Roberts, 2002) and programmes such as Sure Start, Sure Start Plus and Children's Fund are driven by the belief that early and multifaceted intervention results in long-term benefits.

Discussion has focused on variations in outcomes associated with socioeconomic position but other factors are also related to significant differences in health outcomes. For example:

- Babies of mothers born in Pakistan have an infant mortality rate more than double the overall infant mortality rate in the UK.
- The infant mortality rate for teenage mothers is 60 per cent higher than for older mothers (a young woman from social class V is ten times more likely to be teenage mother than a better-off young woman from social class I).
- A large proportion of looked after young people (between 14 per cent (Biehal *et al.*, 1992) and 25 per cent (Garnett, 1992)) have a child by the age of 16, and nearly 50 per cent are mothers within 18 to 24 months after leaving care (Biehal *et al.*, 1995; Corlyon and McGuire, 1997).

In relation to sexual health, initiatives such as the Youth Development Centres being piloted from late 2003 in England have combined efforts to improve sexual health outcomes and to target efforts at those most in need.

The focus of this section

The chapters in this section look at groups who may require special or additional attention. This may be needed because of poorer sexual health outcomes, but also perhaps because of specific support needs and/or inadequate provision by mainstream services. Focusing on certain groups does not mean that the needs of others are less pressing – for example, the issues for young black people as opposed to young Pakistani people. Nor are those who require extra attention necessarily 'marginalized' or members of minority groups – young men have received relatively little attention compared with young women, yet they constitute half of the youth population.

A key issue in relation to supporting those who may have additional or specific needs in relation to sexual health is whether they are better provided for within the mainstream or by specialist services. Current policies focus on inclusion and integration. This might include adapting or extending mainstream services, for example by attaching sexual health services to drugs services for those involved in prostitution, integrating health promotion advice as part of general practice, or providing culturally sensitive health materials and advice in schools.

An advantage of integration is that it can be more resource efficient, can make the linking of health issues easier, and if appropriately done, can avoid reinforcing feelings of exclusion. There is also broader evidence of the effectiveness of addressing sexual health as part of a programme of work rather than as a separate issue. For example, holistic youth development or 'life skills' approaches are showing promising results in the USA with respect to dealing with a range of risky behaviours (Roth *et al.*, 1998; Kirby, 2001; Swann *et al.*, 2003).

However, for some groups or issues there may also be a case for separate provision. Specialist expertise might be needed, or services in specific geographic locations, or even linguistically tailored services. It is important in these cases to avoid the negative labelling or stigmatization that can arise for some groups if they are 'treated differently' (as was the case with AIDS and gay men in the 1980s) and to guard against threats to confidentiality that might arise from young people being seen to attend a specially tailored service.

The ideal is flexibility of response, whether that is mainstream, specialist, or mixed provision. This means listening to the voice of young people and finding out what they are most likely to respond to, something which is even more important when professional knowledge and experience about a group's detailed needs are limited (for example, due to different cultural backgrounds).

This focus on 'giving voice' to users, and working with local communities is a growing issue at national and regional levels. However, it is challenging for professionals, not just to find ways of listening to these views but also to interpret and use them to inform decisions, especially if they are at odds with their own professional expertise or personal beliefs and values. In relation to young people's sexual health such issues, often arising from generational and cultural differences, can be significant.

So there are common issues relating to how best to provide information and support to those who may need additional support in appropriately tailored and targeted ways that take account of user views and broader social and cultural norms. This is often difficult for policy makers and providers, who are constrained by national and local political agendas and by the financial and human resources that they have available. Competition for these resources is inevitable and decisions about priorities are shaped by:

- Evidence of greatest need, although evidence of need for all groups may not be available and even if it is it can be difficult to make comparisons across groups.
- Evidence of likely impact – what interventions are likely to be most effective, even if these address better the needs of some groups whose needs are less acute?
- Strength of advocacy for certain groups or issues, their political salience, and the potential public response to certain courses of action. Public response in particular can be a major factor in whether marginalized minority groups get the attention that they may need, as in the case of support for asylum seekers.

Many of the issues facing young people with respect to improving their sexual health are shared. Regardless of what groups they belong to, the importance of sensitive, confidential and non-judgmental support, offered in ways that reflect an understanding of broader social and cultural factors is clear. However, it is also clear that some groups have been addressed inadequately, and additional attention to their needs is required. Which groups receive priority and on what basis remain key questions.

References

Acheson, D. (1998) *Independent Inquiry into Inequalities in Health*. London: HMSO.

Biehal, N. *et al.* (1992) *Prepared for Living? A Survey of Young People Leaving the Care of the Local Authorities*. London: National Children's Bureau.

Biehal, N. *et al.* (1995) Leaving care in England: a research perspective. *Children and Youth Services Review* **16**: 231–54.

Corlyon, J. and McGuire, C. (1997) *Young Parents in Public Care*. London: National Children's Bureau.

Garnett, L. (1992) *Leaving Care and After*. London: National Children's Bureau.

Kirby, D. (2001) *Emerging Answers: Research Findings on Programs to Reduce Unwanted Teen Pregnancy*. Washington DC: National Campaign to Prevent Teen Pregnancy.

Mielck, A., Graham, H. and Bremberg, S. (2001) Children: an important target group for the reduction of socioeconomic inequalities in health, in J. Mackenbach and M. Bakker (eds), *Reducing Inequalities in Health: A European Perspective*. London: Routledge.

Roberts, H. (2002) Reducing inequalities in child health, in D. McNeish, T. Newman and H. Roberts, *What Works For Children*. Milton Keynes: Open University Press (Barnardo's).

Roth, J., Brooks-Gunn, J., Murray, L. and Foster, W. (1998) Promoting health adolescence: synthesis of youth development program evaluations. *Journal of Research on Adolescence*, **8**(4): 423–59.

Scottish Executive (2003) *Improving Health in Scotland – The Challenge*. Edinburgh: The Stationery Office.

Swann, C., Bowe, K., McCormick, G. and Kosmin, M. (2003) *Teenage Pregnancy and Parenthood: A Review of Reviews*. London: Health Development Agency.

Treasury (2002) *Cross-Cutting Spending Review on Health Inequalities*. London: The Stationery Office.

6 Sex, Pregnancy and Parenthood for Young People who are Looked After by Local Authorities

JUDY CORLYON

Key issues

- Young people looked after often have more health and sex education needs than their peers but appear to receive less attention.
- Many of the needs of looked after young people for information and support regarding relationships and communication go unmet. This appears to be particularly the case for boys and young men.
- Carers and social workers cannot be expected to provide SRE unless they are trained to do so and have clear policies and guidelines within which to work.

Overview

This chapter explores the position of young people looked after by local authorities in terms of their access to information about sex, the reasons for unintentional or planned pregnancy and their experiences of early pregnancy. It highlights how wider aspirations and expectations play a significant role both in the choices these young people make with regard to sexual behaviour and in the issues that practitioners need to address in order to provide adequate support.

Introduction

Any attempt to understand and address the sexual health needs of young people must take account of the broader context of their lives, in which attitudes, expectations and behaviours are shaped. This is particularly so in the case of young people who are 'looked after', or under the formal care of the state.

In 2000 there were around 80,000 children and young people looked after in the UK. This is a diverse group with different issues and needs, and although many do not lead the chaotic lives that are often portrayed in stereotypes, many are affected by disturbed relationships and a discontinuity of care that has implications for health and wellbeing. For example, regarding sexual health specifically, they may miss out on some of the formal structures (close family environments, continuous mainstream schooling) that facilitate effective sex education, and may need additional support as a result (Haydon, 2003). They are also more likely to conceive and become parents at an early age (Social Exclusion Unit, 1999), and the impact of this on them, and their subsequent children, may be different from that on other young people because their lives are often already more challenging.

This chapter explores some of the potential reasons that young people who are looked after get pregnant and become parents, and what these mean for providing adequate information and support. Their general sex information and health needs are also addressed. Although the underlying support needs echo those for young people in general, their emphasis or salience may be different because of particular features in the lives of young people who are looked after. It is also important to note that for some young people parenthood is a deliberate choice that can bring positive aspects.

Young people looked after in the UK

For some children and young people the state assumes a formal role in providing care. Reasons for the state to assume care include serious illness or disability, conviction of a criminal offence demanding a custodial sentence, or inability of a parent to provide appropriate care (often linked to concerns about abuse or neglect). This chapter deals mainly with the last group.

In England and Wales, the Children Act 1989 introduced the term 'looked after' to replace the term 'in care'.[1] Children looked after are those who are placed in the care of local authorities, primarily assigned to foster carers or residential homes, although sometimes remaining in their own homes. They are placed in care either by the courts (under 'care orders') or on a voluntary basis following a request from a parent who is unable to provide the necessary care at home, or from a young person who feels that their domestic circumstances are intolerable.

At March 2002, 59,700 children were looked after in England, of whom:

- 56 per cent were male.
- 41 per cent were aged under 10.
- 64 per cent were under care orders.
- 66 per cent were in foster placements.
- 13 per cent were in children's homes and residential schools.
- 11 per cent were placed with their parents, with social work support.
- 6 per cent were placed for adoption.
  (Source: Department of Health, www.doh.gov.uk/public/cla2002.htm)

Placement in care might be short or long term. Of the 6700 young people aged 16 and over who left care during the year ending 31 March 2002, a quarter had experienced a final period of care of less than a year. Conversely, for nearly two-thirds of the care leavers, their final stay had been for two years or more (www.doh.gov.uk/public/cla2002.htm). However, it should be noted that these figures only reflect the final care episode and not how many times a child or young person has been looked after.

The Children (Scotland) Act 1995 details the responsibilities that Scottish local authorities are required to assume to support vulnerable young people. At March 2002, 11,200 children and young people were being looked after by local authorities in Scotland, of whom:

- 58 per cent were male.
- 52 per cent were under 11.
- 28 per cent were with in foster placements.
- 44 per cent were at home with parents.
- 14 per cent were in residential accommodation (including secure accommodation).

(Source: Scottish Executive National Statistics, Nov 2002 Bulletin www.scotland.gov.uk/stats/bulletins/00199-00.asp)

Unlike in England and Wales, children and young people looked after in Scotland include those under home supervision orders – that is, still living at home – imposed by the Children's Hearings System. This is Scotland's unique system of juvenile justice, set up in 1971 to deal with those under 16 who have committed an offence or are in need of care and protection (in 2000–2001, 32,000 children were referred to this system: NCH, 2003).

Across the UK, older children, and especially teenagers, are more likely to have had a troubled care history with frequent changes of placement, less likely to attract potential adoptive parents, and more likely to live in residential care.

This chapter focuses on young people living in residential care, although there is movement between this and foster care, and many young people will have had experience of both. While many of the issues are similar across the UK, much of the research data and background information is drawn from the English context.

Conception and early pregnancy

Detailed data on rates of teenage conceptions among young women looked after are difficult to obtain, since local authorities have not routinely recorded conceptions among those in their care. However, research indicates that children who have been looked after are around 2.5 times more likely to become teenage parents than those brought up with both natural parents (Social Exclusion Unit, 1999). Between 14 per cent and 25 per cent of young women leave care pregnant or with a child, or have a child shortly after they leave (Biehal *et al.*, 1992; Garnett, 1992). This compares with fewer than 4 per cent of young women in the same age group (under 20) giving birth. Almost half the young women leaving care in a 1995 study were mothers within two years (Biehal *et al.*, 1995).

Experience of the care system in itself can increase vulnerability across many aspects of health. In addition, young people looked after experience more of the other factors directly associated with increased risk of early pregnancy and parenthood. These include: family poverty; low educational attainment, high rates of absenteeism and school exclusion; being without education, training or work at age 16 or 17; sexual abuse; mental health problems; belonging to an ethnic minority (Social Exclusion Unit, 1999). These are explored further below.

Risk and vulnerability

Education

Lack of education is one area where young people who are looked after are probably among the most vulnerable. Truancy and exclusion are major issues. In a study of 48 residential homes, almost a third of those who should have been in school were not (Sinclair and Gibbs, 1998), and national statistics show high rates of non-attendance and increased likelihood of exclusion from school (Department of Health, 1995).

Similarly, there is evidence that young people who are looked after achieve less academically than their peers (Borland *et al.*, 1998). Nearly three-quarters of young people leave care without educational qualifications and very few continue in education beyond the minimum school-leaving age (NCH, 2000; Ritchie, 2003). Lack of qualifications makes securing employment harder, which in turn can lead to a lack of ambition. And teenage parents who are looked after tend to achieve even less academically than other young people who are looked after: 83 per cent of young mothers leaving care had no qualifications compared with 65 per cent of those without children (Biehal *et al.*, 1992).

Instability

Lack of stability is a major problem in the care system. Changes of placement can occur frequently and for a variety of reasons. The original placement might be temporary, especially if it arises out of an emergency, and last only until a permanent one is found. Or the relationship between a foster carer and child might break down, necessitating a move to a new placement with another foster carer or in a residential home. For some children and young people, movement in and out of the care system as family circumstances change is not uncommon. Moreover, placement changes often take place at short notice or fail to happen at the planned time, inevitably producing a further negative impact on the child's sense of security. In the midst of such movement the wishes and preferences of the child or young person might be overlooked, with the result that subsequent placements might be jeopardized.

Relationships

Many young people looked after have difficult or non-existent relationships with parents, especially with fathers, who are more likely than mothers to play no part at all in their lives. The experience of care often does not improve matters: poor relationships tend to stay poor or become worse, and non-existent ones remain so. In some instances carers and social workers are a source of alternative close relationships, but they cannot generate the consistent one-to-one relationships that ideally occur within families. A common complaint of children and young people is that social workers cannot be relied upon to visit frequently or regularly and are generally unavailable when needed. In this way, the feelings of not being cared about are reinforced, and trust and respect appear to be absent from the relationships with significant adults in their lives. Within this void, relationships with peers assume paramount importance: they are the ones who show trust and who respect their ideas. But maintaining friendships can be difficult when lives are disrupted by placement changes.

Health

The poor general health and health care of children and young people who are looked after are a major concern (House of Commons, 1998; Saunders and Broad, 1997). The health care available to them does not always reach the optimum standard. This is partly due to poor inter-departmental and inter-agency working (Department of Health, 1997), which has meant that in some areas medical and social assessments have been carried out separately when clearly the two are inextricably linked (Mather, 2000). Being looked after can also impact on health care because of the disruptive nature of life in general, which can lead to discontinuity of medical care and to erratic patterns of education that mean routine school health checks may be missed.

More specifically, young people who are looked after are more prone to emotional and psychological vulnerability (Richardson and Joughin, 2000). This may be linked to abuse or neglect within the family, which accounted for nearly two-thirds of children who were received into care in 2001/2 in England (Department of Health, 2002). Self-harming behaviours, including suicide attempts, and risky behaviours – drug and alcohol use, unsafe sex practices and sex work – are not uncommon among young people looked after.

Sources of information and support

Under the terms of the Children Act 1989 local authorities in England have duties regarding the sex education of the children and young people they look after. Volume 4 of the accompanying Guidance and Regulations recognizes the likely gap in provision:

> The experience of being cared for should also include the sexual education of the young person. This may, of course, be provided by the young person's school, but if it is not, the SSD or other caring agency responsible for the young person should provide sexual education for him.
>
> (Department of Health, 1991, Section 7.48)

Nevertheless, it is only recently that policies and training for staff have begun to ensure that sex and relationships education (SRE) for young people looked after takes place. Previously there were no policies or practice guidelines, and social workers and carers were typically untrained and thus not able or confident to deliver sex education. They were also often uncertain of the extent of both their own responsibilities and the wishes of parents, especially if placement agreement meetings had not been held. At such meetings all parties involved in the welfare of the child or young people should be present and parental preferences discussed. This provides the opportunity to explore potentially delicate topics, such as how, when and by whom sex education should be provided.

Where there is no such policy on SRE for young people looked after, a potential advantage is that each case can be treated on an individual basis, ideally to meet the best interests of the young person in that situation. However, with a complete lack of guidance the consequent burden of individual discretion placed on those working directly with the young person can prove to be too onerous. Fear of being held responsible can lead to no, or minimal, intervention. Furthermore, workers operating without clear guidelines can find themselves in a difficult position, open to allegations of advocating sexual relations between young people if they encourage the use of contraception but to charges of dereliction of duty if a young woman becomes pregnant.

According to young people in a study by Corlyon and McGuire (1999),[2] inputs from residential carers are minimal, usually consisting of responses to individual questions rather than initiating discussions. However this approach can meet with understanding rather than criticism:

> I think it's actually a bit difficult for care staff to say things at the right time.... I think it's a dodgy situation because there's a lot of tearaways in care that won't listen to anything they've got to say.
>
> [17 year old female]

Despite possible concerns about SRE provision in the care setting, young people there do claim to know about sex and contraception. This may be because, as with their peers in the wider population, they also have access to information through schools, family and friends. For example, schools provide SRE and although there may be issues concerning timing, content and delivery, basic information is available and recent government initiatives are likely to bring improvements (see Chapter 12). However, many children who are looked after are simply not at school and would be missed by even the best provision in that setting.

Parents too may be sources of information and guidance, since some young people only enter the care system in adolescence and might well have had the opportunity for discussion at home (although there is little evidence of this being a frequent occurrence).

However, more usual sources are friends, and information from conversations and magazines. Significantly, although reliable information about sexual health may be difficult to come by, these young people do not consider themselves uninformed. Information may be patchy and incomplete but sufficient to establish a false sense of understanding and to contribute to the increased rates of pregnancy in this group.

Reasons for engaging in sexual relationships

Of course, lack of information is not the only reason that young people looked after make the choices they do regarding sexual behaviour. Many other factors account for reduced use of contraceptive methods and for why teenagers either unintentionally or deliberately become parents, some of which are common to other groups and have been discussed elsewhere in this book.

Pressure between peers and within relationships

Pressure from peers to have sex, either directly or through feelings of wanting to belong or seeking peer approval, is an important issue for many young people. In the wider youth community, it is often girls who are identified as bearing the brunt of this pressure from boys. However, boys who are looked after typically query the girls' assertion that they are the ones who apply pressure, and a substantial number of them believe that the reverse situation applies and that they are the target of pressure from girls (Table 6.1). Yet this is an area on which they have little information. Many girls who are looked

Table 6.1 Pressure to have sex

	Looked after sample (%)		Comparator sample (%)	
	Male	Female	Male	Female
Believes that boys pressurize girls into having sex	34	76	48	75
Believes that girls pressurize boys into having sex	49	18	25	23

Note: Significant difference between males in samples for both beliefs.
Source: Corlyon and McGuire, 1999

after agree that they put pressure on boys to have a girlfriend, but it is unclear whether this involves a sexual relationship or is a symbolic gesture.

Fear of being excluded from a particular group may also be a strong influencing factor on sexual behaviour among those who have experienced rejection and who are seeking approval: in this situation, sleeping with a partner can provide the entry ticket to the group. This is made easier on a practical level because those living in residential care cannot be given the same level of individual supervision typically associated with family life, offering them greater opportunities for behaving as they wish.

Work addressing the issue of peer pressure has tended to focus on issues of communication and negotiation, both strongly linked to self-esteem which in turn is linked with behaviours associated with poor sexual health outcomes. Although the emphasis on self-esteem has not gone unchallenged, a recent study that found low self-esteem may not be as significant as it is often assumed to be in relation to delinquency, violence and educational under-attainment, nevertheless noted that it is a factor in suicide attempts, depression and teenage pregnancy (Emler, 2001).

Feelings of invincibility

Lack of concern or exaggerated feelings of invincibility may make the possibility of pregnancy seem less salient. Young people who are looked after worry less about the possibility of pregnancy than those who are not looked after. The difference is especially marked among the males: more than three-quarters of the looked after boys claim never or only sometimes to worry about whether their girlfriend would become pregnant, and 43 per cent were reportedly too embarrassed to discuss contraception with a new partner. These are both roughly double the rates among their peers who are living with their families (Corlyon and McGuire, 1999).

Intimacy and love

Young people who are looked after tend to embark on relationships at a relatively early age. Having a girlfriend/boyfriend assumes a special significance and is a possible route to feeling valued and loved, especially for those who have already experienced insecurity, loneliness and rejection and who have no sense of belonging:

> Because people in care have such a shitty life they feel better if they're going to bed with someone. They get to feel 'they love me because they sleep with me' but their past has a lot to do with it.
>
> (15 year old female)

Most young people want to be in a steady relationship (not necessarily cohabiting) within four years. But more than half of those who are looked after, significantly more than those living with their families, state that they want to be married or cohabiting and have a child. Table 6.2 shows more boys than girls who are looked after aspire to this early coupledom (80 per cent as opposed to 48 per cent).

Table 6.2 Expectations in relationships and parenthood status ('In four years I would like to ...')

| | Looked after sample (%) | | Comparator sample (%) | |
	Male	Female	Male	Female
Be in a steady relationship with someone	87.5	90	84	89
Be married or living with a boyfriend or girlfriend	80	48	42	38
Have at least one child	55	47	30	17

Note: Significant difference between males in samples on issues two and three
Source: Corlyon and McGuire, 1999

Aspirations and expectations

Lack of care, poor educational qualifications and poor prospects of employment can mark the beginning of a spiral in which pregnancy and motherhood become options which are more attractive than many others. Where young women have low aspirations and feel that there are few opportunities available to them or that they are unable to access alternative means by which to acquire adult identities, parenthood may appear to provide a means by which to become grown up, needed and loved (Musick, 1993; Coleman and Dennison, 1998).

Table 6.3 shows similarities and differences in aspirations: specifically in terms of employment between young people looked after and their peers in the wider community. Looking ahead four years, most want to be in education, training or employment, and there is little difference between the aspirations of teenagers who are looked after and those who are not.

They also identify similar obstacles to obtaining employment, such as lack of qualifications and training and a shortage of jobs. However, 50 per cent of those looked after compared with only 9 per cent of the comparator group envisage that their background will prevent them obtaining a job they would like, and 44 per cent, compared with 12 per cent of those not looked

Table 6.3 Aspirations for future employment
('In four years I would like to ...')

| | Looked after sample (%) | | Comparator sample (%) | |
	Male	Female	Male	Female
Be in a secure job	92	92	84.5	68
Be at college or university (or about to go)	62	83	67	73
Be doing some form of training	65	85	81	71

Note: Significant difference between males in samples on issue three
Source: Corlyon and McGuire, 1999

after, also think that their employment prospects will be damaged by virtue of having been in trouble with the law.

While a greater proportion of boys than girls who are looked after are concerned about the potential effect of criminal activities, the girls are significantly more likely than the boys, and significantly more likely than the girls in the comparator sample, to state that already having a child may affect their employment ambitions (see Table 6.4).

Table 6.4 Factors young people believe prevent them from getting a job they would like

| | Looked after sample (%) | | Comparator sample (%) | |
	Male	Female	Male	Female
Shortage of jobs	49	38.5	49	57
Insufficient qualifications or training	53	46	36	47
Previous offending behaviour	51	36.5	17	15
Being a parent	14	31	17	15

Note: Significant difference between males in samples on issues two and three and between females on issues one, three and four
Source: Corlyon and McGuire, 1999

Breaking the cycle

Parenthood is also seen as a chance to 'set the record straight' and make amends for parents' behaviour. When asked 'What does being a parent mean to you?' 77 per cent of those looked after agree that it meant 'having the chance to do things differently if you have had a bad experience'; this compared with 56 per cent of the comparison group. The looked after group rate showing and telling children you love them as the most important of the aspects of parenthood listed. They also rate giving praise more highly than the comparison group (61 per cent versus 45 per cent).

The teenagers who are looked after, and the girls in particular, are almost twice as likely as those not in care to say they would like to learn more about child care and being a parent. But for those who do become mothers it would appear that much more parenting information and support is required.

Pregnancy as a positive choice

For some care leavers with no qualifications, little income and limited possibility of accommodation, having a baby is one way of demonstrating that they are mature and worthy of the same status as peers who gain qualifications, study in further/higher education, or work. Parenthood may be a positive aspiration for young people with few alternative opportunities.

For others, having a baby may be a source of constancy in a disrupted life; providing some stability and a source of purpose and identity (Mullins and McCluskey, 1999). Young people who are looked after are more likely to choose parenthood in order to have someone to love. Looked after young people of both sexes are often keener to want a baby by the time they are 20 than young people living with their families (51 per cent compared with 24 per cent) (Corlylon and McGuire, 1999). Many perceive parenthood as an opportunity to compensate for their own negative experiences of family relationships and being parented.

Responses to unintended pregnancy

Although for the reasons outlined above pregnancy may be a positive choice for some young people looked after, many pregnancies are unintended and some may be the result of sexual abuse. Such unintended pregnancies can be a cause of immense anxiety and anguish not typically alleviated by carers or parents.

One young woman described her situation thus:

I was absolutely terrified of telling them (care staff) I was pregnant, plus I was scared myself. I told D, the officer in charge, and it took me about ten minutes to tell her and she just turned round and said something like 'stupid bitch'.

Another tried different avenues without success:

> I phoned my mum but it was nothing to do with her because she hadn't
> brought me up and I phoned the baby's father and he said he would come
> down but he didn't.... Then every time I phoned my social worker she
> was out or busy or in a meeting, so I just left it.

'Just leaving it' is a decision-making approach that fits with the experiences
of many young people who are looked after. Because they are unused to
participating in decisions made about their lives, and because decisions made
for them are typically hasty and short term (House of Commons, 1998),
they experience difficulty seeing beyond the immediate future and they
develop a tendency to 'live for the day'. Many young people who are looked
after have difficulty engaging in pragmatic discussions about their future,
making comments such as 'I ain't even thought about what I'm gonna do
tomorrow!' or 'You could get run over by a bus tomorrow, couldn't you?'
Rather than assuming any degree of control, they appear to adopt a fatalis-
tic acceptance of whatever happens to them. This ties in with their approach
to contraceptive use, where the potential consequences of their lack of action
do not weigh too heavily.

Tabberer *et al.* (2000) indicated that few sources of impartial advice are
available for pregnant teenagers. However, they found that the nature of the
advice received and the expectations of family support were critical factors in
the decision about whether to terminate or continue with a pregnancy. Similarly, the young women's own families were crucial in providing ongoing
support and integrating the young women into ordinary family life.

These options are not open to many of the young women looked after
who are pregnant or mothers. In the absence of help from parents, the main
sources of support are most likely to be carers and aftercare workers.
However, a move from residential or foster care into a mother and baby unit,
which ostensibly provides training for independent living, often means there
is no subsequent referral to an aftercare service. As a result these young
mothers are likely to find themselves living in the community, with less
support than their childless peers and less well equipped to deal with decisions than young mothers who have not been looked after.

Conclusion

The reasons why young people who are being or have been looked after are
more likely to experience teenage pregnancy and parenthood are complex,
intertwined and not amenable to easy solutions. However, local authorities
could decrease these young people's vulnerability to unintended pregnancy
and could increase the level of support to those who do become pregnant.

One important step forward would be to ensure that they have some
stability in their lives and are not passed around from one carer to the next.

As a result of this constant movement and the lack of planning in their lives, these young people see the future as a series of short-term interventions based on decisions made by other people. Consequently they have a foreshortened view of the future and operate on a timescale that precludes looking at a period some months ahead.

Many young people who are looked after appear to lack examples of positive relationships and opportunities to learn about trust and respect and, feeling unloved and uncared for, are likely to enter into a relationship without consideration of either the suitability of the partner or the emotional implications of their actions. At practice level it would appear that unless young people are both given genuine affection and helped to understand that it does not have to be contingent upon sex they are likely to continue in their search for love through sexual relationships and parenthood.

Boys and young men who are looked after appear to feel pressure from girls to enter into relationships. At the same time they are unlikely to see prevention of pregnancy as a priority, and are likely to feel too embarrassed to discuss contraception with a new partner. Moreover, they are even more likely than girls who are looked after to aspire to marriage and parenthood at an early age. There is clearly scope, therefore, for more attention to be paid to the communication skills, sex education and emotional needs of these young men.

Living in residential care seems to place extra pressure on young people to embark on sexual relationships at a relatively early age, and to provide them with the opportunities for doing so. More, and more reliable, information about relationships, contraception and pregnancy might help reduce unintended conceptions to young women who are being or have recently been looked after. However, if young people looked after are to receive this information, and if those working with them are to be supported and trained to deliver it, then policies and guidelines on sex and relationships education for them must be in place. Such policies should also incorporate clear courses of action to be followed when young women do become pregnant to ensure that they receive both the support which they need and the facts which will enable them to make an informed decision about the future.

As it is, when they do become pregnant they are often uncomprehending of the long-term implications, unpractised in decision making and unquestioningly accepting of their fate. As a result they are liable to do nothing, which in this case means becoming a teenage parent even when that is not their desired outcome.

Notes

1 The Children Act 1989 was designed primarily for England and Wales with certain provisions applying to Scotland and Northern Ireland. The Children (Scotland) Act 1995 was brought in to extend the Children Act to Scotland with certain differences, for example around children in need. In 1995, the Children (Northern Ireland) Order was passed for the same purpose. Welsh

devolution means separate statutory instruments and regulations are needed to govern devolved issues such as those relating to child care.

2 The quotes, statistics and tables in this chapter are taken from a study by Corlyon and McGuire (1999) into pregnancy and parenthood among looked after young people. Data were collected from 212 young people aged 14 and 15, half of whom were looked after, predominantly in residential care, and half of whom were living with their families, and from 30 pregnant young women and young mothers who were, or had recently been, in the care of a local authority.

References

Biehal, N., Clayden, J., Stein, M. and Wade, J. (1992) *Prepared for Living? A Survey of Young People Leaving the Care of the Local Authorities.* London: National Children's Bureau.

Biehal, N., Clayden, J., Stein, M. and Wade, J. (1995) *Moving On. Young People and Leaving Care Schemes.* London: HMSO.

Borland, M., Pearson, C., Hill, M., Tisdall, K. and Bloomfield, I. (1998) *Education and Care Away From Home.* Edinburgh: Scottish Council for Research in Education.

Coleman, J. and Dennison, C. (1998) Teenage parenthood. *Children and Society* **12**(4): 306–14.

Corlyon, J. and McGuire, C. (1999) *Pregnancy and Parenthood: The Views and Experiences of Young People in Public Care.* London: National Children's Bureau.

Department of Health (1991) The Children Act 1989: Guidance and Regulations. *Volume 4 Residential Care.* London: HMSO.

Department of Health (1995) *The Education of Children who are Looked After by Local Authorities.* London: Department of Health Social Services Inspectorate.

Department of Health (1997) *When Leaving Home is also Leaving Care.* London: The Stationery Office.

Department of Health (2002) www.doh.gov.uk/public/cla2002.htm

Emler, N. (2001) *Self-Esteem: The Costs and Causes of Low Self-Worth.* York: Joseph Rowntree Foundation.

Garnett, L. (1992) *Leaving Care and After.* London: National Children's Bureau.

Haydon, D (2003) *Teenage pregnancy and looked after children/care leavers: resource for teenage pregnancy co-ordinators.* Barnardo's, www.teenagepregnancyunit.gov.uk

House of Commons (1998) *Children Looked After by Local Authorities: Health Committee Second Report.* London: The Stationery Office.

Mather, M. (2000) Health needs of looked after children. *Children's Residential Care Unit Newsletter* **13** (Spring): 3–4.

Moore, S. and Rosenthal, D. (1993) *Sexuality in Adolescence.* London: Routledge.

Mullins, A. and McCluskey, J. (1999) *Teenage Mothers Speak for Themselves.* London: NCH Action for Children.

Musick, J. (1993) *Young, Poor and Pregnant: The Psychology of Teenage Motherhood.* New Haven: Yale University Press.

NCH (2000) *Factfile 2001. Facts and Figures about Children in the UK.* London: NCH.

NCH (2003) *Factfile 2003.* London: NCH.

Richardson, J. and Joughin, C. (2000) *Mental Health Needs of Looked After Children.* London: Gaskell.

Ritchie, A. (2003) *Care to Learn? The Educational Experience of Children and Young People who are Looked After.* Scotland, Glasgow: Save the Children and Who Cares?

Saunders, L. and Broad, B. (1997) *The Health Needs of Young People Leaving Care.* Leicester: De Montfort University.

Sinclair, I. and Gibbs, I. (1998) *Children's Homes: A Study in Diversity.* Chichester: Wiley.

Social Exclusion Unit (1999) *Teenage Pregnancy.* London: The Stationery Office.

Tabberer, S., Hall, C., Prendergast, S. and Webber, A. (2000) *Teenage Pregnancy and Choice: Abortion or Motherhood: Influences on the Decision.* York: Joseph Rowntree Foundation.

7 Addressing the Sexual Health Needs of Young Lesbian, Gay and Bisexual People

KATIE BUSTON

> **Key issues**
>
> - Heterosexism and homophobia, manifested in bullying, abuse and the invisibility of LGB identities, can lead to same-sex attracted young people being reluctant to access relevant sexual health information and advice and to seek help.
> - Heterosexism and homophobia can mean that school sex education and sexual health services do not cater adequately to the needs of this group.
> - Inclusivity should be the guiding principle of education and health-care provision, and heterosexism and homophobia should be challenged at all levels.

Overview

This chapter examines the sexual health needs of lesbian, gay and bisexual (LGB) young people in the UK, exploring the impact of the heterosexist culture in which they grow up. It focuses on school sex education, sexual health services and alternative models of service provision, and presents examples of promising practice.

Introduction

Although existing data sources do not provide good information about sexual orientation and associated needs, it is known that a significant minority of young people in the UK have same-sex feelings. Some will have engaged in same-sex sexual activity and/or will identify as lesbian, gay and bisexual (LGB).

LGB youth are as diverse as heterosexual youth (Savin-Williams, 2001), spanning ethnic and social class groupings and different areas of the country. There are also significant differences within the LGB group, in patterns of attitudes and behaviours and in sexual health needs. However, there are areas of commonality and mutual interest, in particular around exclusion, discrimination and stigma, and it is reasonable to address the main issues for the whole group, although much of the research, policy and practice focuses on gay men in particular, and to a much lesser extent lesbians.

Historically, the needs of young LGB people have tended to be constructed in physical terms, as illustrated by the response to the predicted HIV/AIDS pandemic in the 1980s, which resulted in a raft of education, health, community and media interventions aimed mainly at changing the behaviour patterns of gay men. A sustained effort to encourage behaviour change remains vital, since most HIV infection in young people in the UK is a result of unprotected sex between males, and a 1999 survey of gay men showed that 58 per cent of those under 20 engaging in anal intercourse did not always use a condom (Weatherburn *et al.*, 2000). However, a focus on HIV-related work overlooks the physical health needs of lesbians (Douglas *et al.*, 1997; Farquhar *et al.*, 2001) who, although they may have one of the lowest rates of STIs such as gonorrhoea, chlamydia and syphilis, have a relatively high prevalence of viral STIs such as herpes simplex and human papilloma virus (Ford and Clarke, 1998). Moreover, the focus on physical health that grew out of concerns about HIV downplayed important psychological and emotional aspects of sexuality, for example around issues of discrimination and stigma.

General moves towards a more inclusive and holistic approach to health and wellbeing have improved the scope and the quality of sexual health work with LGB groups. However, there are still many gaps in knowledge and provision, particularly in relation to the needs of transgender youth. It is known that not all transgender young people are attracted to others of the same sex and that regardless of sexual orientation they face similar issues as LGB groups in terms of access to appropriate services. However, since data about the needs of transgender youth is especially lacking, this chapter will not address this group specifically.

Policy and legislative context

A range of equality and inclusion strategies since the mid-1990s has brought greater attention to the needs of LGB people. However, some subgroups are less visible than others in policy terms, and various barriers to the development of effective support and services remain.

In England and Wales, Section 28 of the 1988 Local Government Act prohibits local authorities from 'intentionally promoting homosexuality'. This has been identified as discriminatory and a reflection of broader heterosexist and homophobic attitudes (Douglas *et al.*, 1997; Scottish Executive, 1999; Buston and Hart, 2001). Attempts to repeal Section 28 were blocked by the House of Lords in July 2000, though more recently the House has voted to repeal the act. While no local authority has ever been charged or prosecuted under Section 28, the legislation is 'a clear signal that there may be something dangerous or wrong about addressing the needs of lesbian, gay or bisexual pupils' (Douglas *et al.*, 1997: 67) and sends a confusing message to teachers which adversely affects their work in delivering inclusive sex education and tackling homophobic bullying.

More legislative progress has been made in Scotland, where the equivalent Section 2a of the 1986 Local Government Act was repealed in 2000, although only after protracted arguments reflected in and fuelled by the media, which uncovered some extreme and negative attitudes towards LGB groups. The consultation paper issued by the Scottish Executive proposing the repeal of Section 2a stated that the original legislation:

> served to legitimise intolerance and prejudice and, arguably, to raise the level of homophobia; acted as an unhelpful constraint on the ability of local authorities to develop best practice in sex education and bullying; and constrained the ability of local authorities to provide grants or funds to gay and lesbian groups in the community.
>
> (Scottish Executive, 1999: 6)

Across all UK regions, the equalization of the age of consent represents a positive development. Prior to June 2001, the age of sexual consent for heterosexuals was 16 years (17 in Northern Ireland) compared with 18 years for homosexuals. This was rectified in 2001 and the age of consent is now 16 years for all (17 years in Northern Ireland). However, again there was considerable resistance to these changes, which were pushed through using a Parliament Act when obstructed by the House of Lords.

Other recent legal and policy changes in the UK include:

- The laws on adoption have changed so that same-sex couples are now able to adopt children on the same basis as heterosexual couples.
- Employment law has been negotiated and the UK has signed up to the European Employment Directive to protect against sacking on the basis of sexual orientation.
- Immigration rules have changed to ensure that a partner from overseas can live in the UK on the basis of a same-sex relationship.
- The Human Rights Act has been introduced, giving protection in the domestic courts from discrimination on the grounds of sexual orientation.
- Guidance has been issued to schools to encourage them to confront homophobic bullying.
- Following a European ruling, the ban on LGB people serving in the armed forces has been lifted.
- The Wales Act and Scotland Act and the Greater London Authority Act carry new powers to promote equality and challenge sexual orientation discrimination.

These changes are positive in terms of greater equity between heterosexual and LGB groups. However, the degree of resistance and the fierceness of debate in relation to some of the changes reflect continuing high levels of heterosexism and homophobia, and some areas remain ripe for reform. For example, there is still no legal recognition of same-sex partnerships, meaning that same-sex couples have no pension rights and have no status as next of kin in the event of the death of one partner. A recent government consultation paper has, however, put forward a proposal which would grant these rights to same-sex couples if they register their partnership in a civil ceremony.

Homophobia and heterosexism: manifestations and impacts

Many of the difficulties faced by LGB young people arise because of homophobia and heterosexism. Homophobia has been defined as 'negative and/or fearful attitudes about homosexuals or homosexuality' (Sprecher and McKinney, 1993: 21). Heterosexism is 'an underlying belief that heterosexuality is the natural/normal/acceptable or superior form of sexuality' (Williamson, 2000: 98).

Whereas homophobia may manifest itself in abuse directed towards those who are, or are perceived to be, attracted to others of the same sex, heterosexism may lead to a presumption that everyone is heterosexual and, more than that, that everyone should be heterosexual. As a result, many young people learn that 'being heterosexual' is the only way to be, with alternative feelings, identities or behaviour regarded as perverse and having to be accounted for (Epstein and Johnson, 1994).

In some groups the norm of opposite-sex attraction may be even stronger and the cost of breaking this norm greater. For example, in black and minority ethnic communities, coming out may bring marginalization or expulsion from groups in which racial solidarity is usually high (Epstein and Johnson, 1994). Experiences are also likely to differ by social class (Flowers and Buston, 2001).

Many young LGB people show great resilience in the face of heterosexism and homophobia (see Meyer and Dean, 1998; Savin-Williams, 2001). However, for many there is a wide range of detrimental effects which can include fear of being 'found out', denial of true feelings, shame, isolation and exclusion, school absenteeism, and even self-harm and suicidal ideation or behaviour (see Frankham, 1996; Rivers, 1997, 2000; Flowers and Buston, 2001; Coia *et al.*, 2002).

Media representations

The dominance of opposite-sex relationships in the media and the relative lack of positive images of alternative sexual orientations (Burton, 1995; Batchelor and Kitzinger, 1999; Flowers and Buston, 2001) may bolster heterosexism or even endorse or encourage homophobia. Soap operas and drama series are often filled exclusively with people who are attracted to the opposite sex, with young people nearly always portrayed as heterosexual. References to lesbianism are often made with a male focus and for titillation, whereas references to male homosexuality often invoke fear or humour (Batchelor and Kitzinger, 1999). The myth that if a gay man meets the right woman he will be 'cured', with his same-sex desires just a stage that he was destined to pass through, is also carried through into media representations (for example, in *Bob and Rose*, a comedy-drama featuring a gay man as the main male character, Bob fell in love with Rose).

Lack of role models

Whereas for many minority groups role models may be scarce in mainstream media, they are available within the school, family and other social spaces. The LGB young person may, however, find it difficult to identify others who are having similar experiences (Flowers and Buston, 2001). As Daniel, a gay man cited by Flowers and Buston (2001: 57) said:

> I could never see that you could be gay here. I thought it was something you would have to go to America to be.

Bullying and abuse

The majority of LGB young people have experienced homophobic abuse and/or violence (Mason and Palmer, 1996; Coia *et al.*, 2002). They may experience rejection and abuse in the home, particularly if they 'come out' to parents and siblings (see Rogers, 1994; Mason and Palmer, 1996; Flowers and Buston, 2001). They may also experience a lack of support from family with regard to bullying taking place elsewhere (Rivers, 1996), because of homophobic attitudes within the family or because attempts to hide their feelings or identity from family members mean they feel unable to share what has been happening to them (see Frankham, 1996).

Bullying and abuse in schools is well documented. For example, Mason and Palmer (1996) found that 48 per cent of the young lesbians and gay men they questioned reported having experienced violence, with 40 per cent of attacks taking place in school, and Rivers (1996) found that 80 per cent of those he questioned reported being called names at school. As well as verbal abuse, the young people taking part in Rivers' (1996) study described having clothes set alight, being urinated upon, and being dragged along by the hair. Few reported seeking support from a teacher (Rivers, 2000). Indeed, Rivers (1995) found that around half of those surveyed recalled being bullied by a teacher because of their actual or perceived sexual orientation. Buston and Hart (2001) describe instances of overt homophobia exhibited by teachers during sex education lessons, including equating paedophilia with homosexuality and using language to problematize homosexuality (for example: 'it's difficult for normal men to be friends with gays' (Buston and Hart, 2001: 100). Flowers and Buston (2001) note that such bullying and abuse can lead fellow pupils and former friends to avoid any association with the victim, worried about being 'tarred with the same brush' (see also Rivers, 1997).

Box 7.1 shows comments made by young people in the SHARE sex education study of 25 Scottish schools between 1996 and 1999 (see Buston and Hart, 2001; Wight *et al.*, 2002). Each focuses on a potential consequence of homophobia and/or heterosexism, providing 'real-life' examples of what growing up identifying as lesbian or gay can mean to individuals. These young people describe school generally, sex education specifically, and/or societal attitudes as failing them and/or people they know.

Box 7.1 Quotes from young people participating in the SHARE sex education study

I think that there must be many people at high school who are either lesbian gay or bisexual but because of the way that LGB people are looked upon by society in general they are unable to ask questions or discuss their thoughts and feelings with friends, parents, or teachers for fear of people 'finding out'. Being gay and going to the school I did was very hard and it made me feel extremely isolated and very very different. I think that in the future (as in the very near future) sex education in school should include educating LG&B people. It should be made clear that there is help for people like myself as I have endured far too many identity crises due to the severe lack of support.

(female, 16 years old)

I feel that sex education was ... not very helpful to me because we never got info or advice about gay relationships.

(female, 16 years old)

With the amount of sick homophobic attitudes this society is plagued with, anyone wanting to come out about their sexuality at our age can't. As a regular Internet user I have met, and continue to speak to many guys my age who are gay – any more of what is said at school about homosexuals and they will want to top themselves. They are scared about coming out and being rejected. Something has to be done before any more gay teenagers commit suicide, the sooner the better. It's discrimination.

(male, 16 years old)

The response of schools to homophobic bullying has been mixed (see Frankham, 1996). In a survey of English schools Warwick *et al.* (2001) found that while 82 per cent of the teachers surveyed were aware of instances of homophobic verbal bullying and 26 per cent were aware of instances of homophobic physical bullying, only 6 per cent of the schools had a bullying policy which made mention of bullying relating to sexual orientation. This was despite 99 per cent of schools having a policy on bullying or discipline, a number of which had specific guidance and methods for addressing racist bullying. In the majority of schools information on support for lesbian and gay pupils was, according to respondents, unavailable. Staff were unsure about how best to address homophobic bullying and parental disapproval, a lack of experienced staff, and a lack of policy were identified by teachers as barriers to tackling it (Warwick *et al.*, 2001). Interestingly, the first exclusively LGB secondary school has just opened in the United States. In receipt of state funding, it has around 100 pupils.

Information and support for young LGB people

All young people have the right to information which they can use to make decisions regarding their relationships and/or sexual behaviour. Regardless of their sexual orientation they experience many of the same dilemmas as they form, or think about forming, romantic and sexual relationships. However, some issues may be particularly salient or stressful to subsections of LGB youth, particularly around coming out. Those who are 'out' often feel relieved that they have confirmed their identity with family and others, and are likely to be more willing, and more able, to access relevant sexual health information (Frankham, 1996). For those who are loathe to admit their feelings even to themselves, or for whom publicly acknowledging these feelings is risky, seeking out information and support is more difficult.

While there is certainly a place for specialist services that are open to or designed especially for particular (and sometimes marginalized) groups of young people, provision as a whole should be inclusive, and when the audience or client base is likely to be diverse (for example, a school class or a general practitioner's surgery), care should be taken to cater for all young people, whatever their sexual identity or background. Teachers, health care professionals and others in contact with young people may need training to ensure that they feel equipped to adopt an inclusive approach, and structural or policy changes at the level of the whole school, whole clinic and so on may be required to facilitate good practice.

Of course, inclusive sex education and sexual health service provision cannot compensate for homophobia and heterosexism elsewhere in society, and it is important that this general climate is also tackled in order to support young LGB people effectively.

School-based sex education

Although there has been little recent systematic research examining what young lesbians and gay men think about the school sex education they have received, earlier research suggests that provision has been inadequate (Mac an Ghaill, 1991; Rogers, 1994; Frankham, 1996). Recent work observing sex education lessons and surveying and interviewing teachers and senior management has shed light on why this may be the case. Buston and Hart (2001) observed sex education lessons delivered by 40 teachers. They found that the lessons of some teachers were inclusive, but others rendered lesbian and gay sexuality invisible or even contained instances of explicit homophobia. Examples of heterosexist or homophobic practice included talking about sexual relationships solely in terms of male/female sex, defining sexual activity solely as penetrative vaginal intercourse; teacher complicity with the homophobic comments of some pupils; teachers teasing boys about 'being gay'; and the use of language by teachers to problematize homosexuality. Conversely, in lessons categorized as 'good practice', homosexuality was normalized alongside heterosexuality and information was given to all pupils as a matter of course, while homophobic comments made by pupils were challenged.

In Warwick *et al.*'s (2001) study, while 51 per cent of the 307 schools surveyed had a policy on sex education which mentioned lesbian and gay related issues, over a third of teachers questioned believed that it was not appropriate to provide such information in schools. When schools did state that they addressed lesbian and/or gay issues in the curriculum it was often only in the context of HIV and AIDS. As well as issues relating to the existence of Section 2a, other barriers to the delivery of inclusive sex education identified by teachers include worries about disruption caused by negative reactions from pupils to inclusive lessons; worries over 'neutrality' (which is generally seen by teachers as important in the delivery of sex education); perceived lack of support and restrictions from senior management; and individual discomfort and prejudice (Buston and Hart, 2001).

Sexual health services

A recent study of young LGB people in Glasgow found that few respondents had encountered difficulties with general practitioner services because of their sexuality (Coia *et al.*, 2002). There is, however, little research on young LGB people's experience of health care. A greater number of studies have focused on the quality and appropriateness of services for lesbians and gay men, with findings less positive than those of Coia *et al.* (2002). Work has pointed to the existence of prejudice (Rose, 1993; Rose, 1994; Farquhar *et al.*, 2001) and ignorance (Brogan, 1997) about same-sex sexuality, which can lead to insensitivity and/or inadequate consideration of the sexual (and other) health needs of clients. As a result, some gay men and lesbians may be loath to access health care or, when

---

Box 7.2 Good practice school sex education

Do:

- begin with relationships, respect and difference, taking up questions of reproduction along the way
- provide information about same-sex sexuality in an integral manner throughout
- acknowledge homosexuality as a valid emotional orientation (and not solely a form of sexual behaviour)
- use inclusive language
- challenge homophobic comments and behaviour and deem them unacceptable
- mirror inclusive classroom approaches in whole school equal opportunity and anti-discrimination policies.

Don't:

- presume all pupils are heterosexual
- define sex simply in terms of heterosexual vaginal penetration and reproduction
- problematize LGB issues.

Sources: Epstein and Johnson (1994); Patrick and Sanders (1994); Rogers (1994); Burton (1995); Frankham (1996); Biddulph (1998); Buston and Hart (2001).

---

they do, may not disclose their identity or intended or actual sexual behaviour to health care professionals (Farquhar *et al.*, 2001). For example, Zeidenstein (1990) cites one woman who reported having a diaphragm fitted simply because she felt unable to tell her GP that she had no need for contraception. Those who do attend and are open about their status may be given inaccurate information. Appropriate advice and care for lesbian clients is often unavailable (Farquhar *et al.*, 2001). Women describing themselves as lesbians are sometimes told that they do not need cervical smears despite there being a range of factors, including smoking and sex with men (which most adult lesbians have experienced), which have been shown to be related to increased risk of abnormal smears and cervical cancer (Farquhar *et al.*, 2001).

Work undertaken with young people in general suggests that they can be reluctant to use health services, particularly in relation to concerns about sexual health, because of perceptions of access and availability and worries about confidentiality (Macfarlane and McPherson, 1995; Oppong-Odiseng and Heycock, 1997; Jacobsen *et al.*, 2000). Particular barriers based on homophobia or heterosexism may mean that some LGB young people are doubly reluctant to seek health care or, if it is sought, to discuss sexual health issues, particularly if they perceive a need to reveal their sexual orientation or behaviour. Young LGB men and women living in small rural communities, where issues of confidentiality and surveillance may be heightened, may find it particularly difficult to approach health services for care or advice on some matters. Indeed, opportunities for access to appropriate information and support are likely to be much more limited in such areas.

As well as work carried out directly by the statutory sector, community-based and voluntary sector work (mainly funded by the statutory sector) is common. Groups concerned with gay men's health have been more successful in attracting funding than groups concerned with other aspects of LGB health, not least because of the perceived greater public health risk relating to HIV/AIDS. For example, Gay Men's Health is funded by Lothian Health Board in Edinburgh and offers a counselling and support service for gay men, free condoms and lubricant, and peer education in gay bars and on the internet. The sense of solidarity among gay men in particular may help such community-led approaches to address the issues effectively in an appropriate and sensitive way, and to engage in work that would be difficult for many statutory bodies because of the public sensitivity to work in this area.

Box 7.3 Good practice sexual health provision

Do:

- eliminate fears of discrimination based on sexual identity/behaviour
- ensure providers are aware of and understand issues salient to same-sex attracted youth and sub-sections of this diverse group
- ensure provision is relevant to individuals whatever their identity and/or sexual behaviour
- pay attention to confidentiality: make sure young people are aware that whoever they are, and whatever the problems they are seeking help for, confidentiality will be paramount
- adopt non-judgmental approaches at all times
- use inclusive language.

Don't:

- presume client is heterosexual
- ask questions which assume that a client is of a particular orientation or that particular behaviours have been or will be engaged in.

Sources: Gruskin (1999); Farquhar *et al.* (2001)

Recent initiatives: a positive future?

Local and national initiatives are increasingly recognizing the discrimination faced by LGB youth and are seeking to change broader social attitudes.

Beyond Barriers is a Scotland-wide initiative designed to challenge prejudice and homophobia and to build links between minority and majority groups. It is funded for three years, from mid-2001, by the Community Fund (formerly the National Lottery Charities Board), and is being run by Stonewall Scotland, Outright Scotland, the Equality Network, and the Stonewall Youth Project. The project provides information, training, research and capacity building skills to groups and organizations in the public, private and voluntary sectors. It has three aims:

- to enable LGB people (and transgender people) to gain the knowledge and skills to develop a more effective community infrastructure within the wider society
- to ensure that local support and services exist and are publicized so that LGB people, particularly in isolated areas, can live their lives free from discrimination and exclusion
- to make 'equality of opportunity' widely recognized as a principle that must come to apply to all people in Scottish society.

Citizenship 21 is a national-level initiative based in London, set up by Stonewall with support from the Community Fund. Its remit is to promote equality and challenge prejudice. It is able to support community projects from across England to enable them to work in partnership and implement projects that challenge prejudice and discrimination against minority groups. Projects funded include a Leeds-based initiative on training in lesbian health for local service providers, and 'Web Works Wonders', a project funding young people in Holloway to set up a website challenging homophobia and racism.

The Stonewall Youth Project, based in Edinburgh, offers information and support on issues and concerns about sexuality, sexual health, mental health and personal relationships to young LBG people. Subgroups include the Stonewall Girlz group for young women, providing a space where young women can meet relatively safely to socialize as well as to discuss particular needs and issues without the agenda of young gay men dominating.

While the existence of such projects is a positive development, a recent study of the views of representatives of LGB organizations in Scotland noted that while statutory funding may be awarded from time to time for the kinds of projects described above, it was generally short term or one-off, making it difficult to develop sustainable provision (McLean and O'Connor, 2003).

Conclusion

This chapter has described the heterosexist and homophobic context experienced by many LGB young people in the UK. Heterosexism and homophobia, manifested in bullying, abuse and the invisibility of LGB identities, can lead to reluctance to access relevant sexual health information and advice and to seek help. Heterosexism and homophobia can also mean that the information and service support that is provided does not cater adequately to the needs of this group. Bad practice continues in some schools, general practices and other institutions: from failing to acknowledge the diversity amongst young people in terms of sexuality, to stigmatizing homosexual identities and/or providing information without considering the particular needs of subsections of young people (for example, young men who are, or who are likely in the future, to practise penetrative sex with other men).

Recent policy and practice initiatives suggest that strides are beginning to be made in ensuring that homophobia and heterosexism are challenged and that the sexual health needs of same-sex-attracted young people are met with inclusivity as the guiding principle. However, there are still significant gaps in basic knowledge about the sexual health needs of some groups (for example, transgender young people) and differences remain in the relative attention given to subgroups in terms of information and service provision (for example, gay men versus lesbians).

References

Batchelor, S. and Kitzinger, J. (1999) *Teenage Sexuality in the Media*. Edinburgh: Health Education Board for Scotland.

Biddulph, M. (1998) Teaching sex and relationships education in secondary schools. *Sex Education Matters* 16:1–8.

Brogan, M. (1997) Healthcare for lesbians: attitudes and experiences. *Nursing Standard* 11: 39–42.

Burton, A. M. (1995) Things that could make a difference: integrating lesbian and gay issues in secondary schools. *Health Education* 5: 20–5.

Buston, K. and Hart, G. (2001) Heterosexism and homophobia in Scottish school sex education: exploring the nature of the problem. *Journal of Adolescence* 24(1) Feb: 95–109.

Coia, N., John, S., Dobbie, F., Bruce, S., McGranachan, M. and Simons, L. (2002) *'Something to Tell You'. A Health Needs Assessment of Young Gay, Lesbian and Bisexual People in Glasgow*. Glasgow: Greater Glasgow Health Board.

Douglas, N., Warwick, I., Kemp, S. and Whitty, G. (1997) *Playing it Safe: Responses of Secondary School Teachers to Lesbian, Gay and Bisexual Pupils, Bullying, HIV and AIDS Education and Section 28*. University of London: Health and Education Research Unit.

Elford, J. (1997) HIV and AIDS in adolescence: epidemiology, in L. Sher (ed.), *AIDS and Adolescents*. Amsterdam: Harwood Academic.

Epstein, D. and Johnson, R. (1994) On the straight and narrow: the heterosexual presumption, homophobias and schools, in D. Epstein and R. Johnson (eds), *Challenging Lesbian and Gay Inequalities in Education*. Buckingham: Open University Press.

Farquhar, C., Bailey, J. and Whittaker, D. (2001) *Are Lesbians Sexually Healthy?*

A Report of the 'Lesbian Sexual Behaviour and Health Survey'. London: South Bank University.

Flowers, P. and Buston, K. (2001) 'I was terrified of being different': exploring gay men's accounts of growing-up in a heterosexist society. *Journal of Adolescence* **24**: 51–65.

Ford, C. and Clarke, K. (1998) Sexually transmitted infections in women who have sex with women: surveillance data should include this category of women. *British Medical Journal* **316**: 556–7.

Frankham, J. (1996) *Young Gay Men and HIV Infection*. Horsham: AVERT.

Gruskin, E. P. (1999) *Treating Lesbians and Bisexual Women*. Thousand Oaks: Sage.

Jacobsen, L. D., Mellanby, A. R., Donovan, B., Taylor, J. H., Tripp, J. and members of the Adolescent Working Group, RCGP (2000) Teenagers' views on general practice consultations and other medical advice. *Family Practice* **17**: 156–8.

Mac an Ghaill, M. (1991) Schooling, Sexuality and male power: towards an emancipatory curriculum. *Gender and Education* **3**: 291–309.

Macfarlane, A. and McPherson, A. (1995) Primary health care and adolescence. *British Medical Journal* **311**: 825–6.

Mason, A. and Palmer, A. (1996) *Queer Bashing. A National Survey of Hate Crimes against Lesbians and Gay Men*. London: Stonewall.

McLean, C. and O'Connor, W. (2003) *Sexual Orientation Research Phase 2: The Future of LGBT Research – Perspectives of Community Organisations*. London: Scottish Executive Social Research.

Meyer, I. and Dean, L. (1998) Internalised homophobia, intimacy and sexual behaviour among gay and bisexual men, in G. Herek (ed.), *Stigma and Sexual Orientation*. Thousand Oaks: Sage.

Oppong-Odiseng, A. and Heycock, E. (1997) Adolescent health services – through their eyes. *Archives of Disease in Childhood* **77**: 115–19.

Patrick, P. and Sanders, S. A. L. (1994) Lesbian and gay issues in the curriculum, in D. Epstein and R. Johnson (eds), *Challenging Lesbian and Gay Inequalities in Education*. Buckingham: Open University Press.

Rivers, I. (1995) The victimisation of gay teenagers in schools: homophobia in education. *Pastoral Care*, March: 35–41.

Rivers, I. (1996) Young, gay and bullied. *Young People Now*, January: 18–19.

Rivers, I. (1997) Violence against lesbian and gay youth and its impact, in M. Schneider (ed.) *Pride and Prejudice: Working with Gay, Lesbian and Bisexual Youth*. Toronto: Central Toronto Youth Services.

Rivers, I. (2000) Social exclusion, absenteeism and sexual minority youth. *Support for Learning* **15**: 3–18.

Rogers, M. (1994) Growing up lesbian: the role of the school, in D. Epstein (ed.), *Challenging Lesbian and Gay Inequalities in Education*. Buckingham: Open University Press.

Rose, L. (1994) Homophobia among doctors. *British Medical Journal* **308**: 586–7.

Rose, P. (1993) Out in the open? *Nursing Times* **89**: 50–2.

Scottish Executive (1999) *Consultation on the Ethical Standards in Public Life etc. (Scotland) Bill*. Edinburgh: Scottish Executive.

Savin-Williams, R. C. (2001) A critique of research on sexual-minority youths.

Journal of Adolescence **24**: 5–13.

Sprecher, S. and McKinney, K. (1993) *Sexuality*. Thousand Oaks: Sage.

Warwick, I., Aggleton, P. and Douglas, N. (2001) Playing it safe: addressing the emotional and physical health of lesbian and gay pupils in the UK. *Journal of Adolescence* **24**: 129–40.

Weatherburn, P., Stephens, M., Reid, D., Hickson, F., Henderson, L. and Brown, D. (2000) *Vital Statistics: Findings from the National Gay Men's Sex Survey 1999*. London: Sigma Research.

Wight, D., Raab, G., Henderson, M., Abraham, C., Buston, K., Hart, G. and Scott, S. (2002) Limits of teacher delivered sex education: interim behavioural outcomes from a randomised trial. *British Medical Journal* **324**, 15 June: 1430–5.

Williamson, I. R. (2000) Internalized homophobia and health issues affecting lesbians and gay men. *Health Education Research: Theory and Practice* **15**: 97–107.

Zeidenstein, L. (1990) Gynaecological and childbearing needs of lesbians. *Journal of Nurse-Midwifery* **35**: 10–18.

8 Service Provision for Meeting the Sexual Health Needs of Young People from Indian, Pakistani and Bangladeshi Communities

HANSA PATEL-KANWAL, OBE

> **Key issues**
>
> - Religious and cultural issues have a significant impact on the sexual health of young people from Indian, Pakistani and Bangladeshi communities. They need to be addressed as part of any service provision response for these communities.
> - Access to information and service provision needs to address the diversity within and between these groups of young people. Young people from these communities need particular reassurance that service providers will maintain confidentiality.
> - Working in partnership can facilitate skills exchange and capacity building between mainstream and targeted service provision. It serves to enhance the quality of sexual health information and services for these young people.

Overview

This chapter addresses the sexual health needs of young people from Indian, Pakistani and Bangladeshi communities and how service providers can respond to these. It highlights the importance of the cultural and religious context that young people from these communities experience, identifying barriers to improving sexual health. It then suggests a range of actions at different levels that could improve access to services and information.

Introduction

The challenge of writing a single chapter on the sexual health needs of young people from Indian, Pakistani and Bangladeshi communities is formidable if the diversity amongst this audience is to be reflected accurately. However, it is possible to explore some of the key issues that impact upon these young people in their struggle to access culturally and linguis-

128

tically appropriate sexual health information, advice and services. The impact of the broader culture within which young people from these communities grow up is important, as is the specific religious and cultural contexts of their families and immediate communities. In addition, conflicts about the values and norms in these cultures can create further difficulties for these young people.

Cultural and religious context

Discussions about sex and sexual health are considered to be culturally taboo issues within these communities. It is rare for these topics to be discussed in public, in mixed gender settings or across generations. So many young people may not have the opportunity to talk about these matters with parents or carers in an open and confident manner.

> There is no way that I could talk about sex at home. If there is any sex on television, my Mum changes the channel, tells me to change it or leaves the room if my Dad is there.
>
> (Indian young woman, aged 17)

Traditionally Indian, Pakistani and Bangladeshi communities expect young men and women to be virgins when they marry. These communities adhere to the concept of '*izzat*' or 'honour' within the family and wider community. Therefore, within this context any 'private', that is, sexual, behaviour disclosed within a public domain is considered to bring 'shame' or '*sharam*' onto the family and the wider community. Consequently, both young men and women may go to extraordinary lengths to ensure that their parents, carers or other community members do not inadvertently discover any premarital or extramarital sexual activity.

Due to these cultural expectations around their behaviour in public, it may not be possible for young people from these communities to openly seek sexual health information and support for fear of being judged by both service providers and their communities.

Within Indian, Pakistani and Bangladeshi communities religion is often interpreted as being inextricably linked to culture, and used to establish norms around sexual behaviour for both men and women.

The protection of virginity is particularly pertinent for women within these communities, and the chaperoning of young women is taken very seriously to ensure that family honour is maintained. In practice there is often a greater degree of flexibility and tacit acceptance around the premarital and extramarital sexual behaviour of young men within Indian, Pakistani and Bangladeshi communities. This also reflects the norms in many other communities around male sexual behaviour, and the double standards that are perceived to exist between the genders. As with many other communities, women are considered to be the moral custodians and carry the responsibility of ensuring that moral values are passed onto the children and young people within their respective families.

Many young people in Indian, Pakistani and Bangladeshi communities have arranged or facilitated marriages where their potential marriage partner is introduced to them by their family or friends. Some parents and carers take the view that learning about sexual matters can be delayed until the young person is ready for marriage, and they can then access the information that they may need at that stage in their development as adults. It is considered unnecessary to provide such information any earlier as 'they will have no use for it and it only serves as a corrupting influence' as one parent said when being consulted about sex and relationships education at their child's school.

It is the expectation within all these communities that following marriage the couple will choose to have children and continue the family heritage. Couples who choose not to have children or are unable to have them may face considerable pressure from families in the form of intrusive questioning why reproduction has not taken place.

As with many other communities, heterosexuality is perceived to be the norm within Indian, Pakistani and Bangladeshi communities. It is therefore a major challenge for gay, lesbian, bisexual and transgendered young people to express their sexualities openly and confidently. These terms are also considered to be western political constructs, and cannot be positively translated into the languages spoken by these communities. Some young people do choose to 'come out', and may experience the range of reactions that young people from other communities face. Where some parents and carers are accepting of the young person, some may be verbally or physically violent and rejecting, and others may choose to ignore what is happening and proceed with the notion that as soon as 'you are married and have children you will be fine'. This level of denial obviously leads to a lot of internal and external conflict within individuals and within their families.

As younger people elect to adopt the norms of the dominant, more liberal 'British' culture, some older people from these communities may feel that community values are being eroded and challenged, and may struggle to try to maintain these because they fear that their young people will lose a positive element of their identity. This can lead to conflicts between parents, other extended family members and young people.

This acceptance of openness about sex and sexuality is even more difficult for first-generation Indian, Pakistani and Bangladeshi communities, and again this has an impact in the home where first and subsequent generations interact. Equally, asylum seeking people from within these communities may initially be very shocked with the degree of openness within this society around sexual health issues and the positive encouragement given to young people from their own communities to discuss such matters openly and honestly: 'When I first came to this country I was so shocked at how open the women were about sex. It was so different back home' (Pakistani parent).

Notwithstanding wider cultural norms and pressures, some parents recognize their children's needs and the influence of the wider society in which their children are developing. In response to this they are becoming more open to young peoples' sexuality, and adopt more pragmatic approaches to parenting. These parents accept that times are changing and that helping their children to 'keep safe' through accessing culturally and linguistically appropriate sexual health information is probably the best way to respond. Yet even when parents are supportive and open in this way, the lack of good quality information and service provision compromises their ability to fully support their children. Ways to address this are explored later in this chapter.

Sexual health of young people from Indian, Pakistani and Bangladeshi communities

Many young Indian, Pakistani and Bangladeshi young people live in deprived areas and experience all the social and economic inequalities associated with this. They are disproportionately represented among those who are excluded from school, are in public care/looked after, and are in young offender institutions. They are also vulnerable to racial discrimination, language and cultural barriers, which prevent them from accessing relevant information and services in general. Given this context, sexual health may not assume a high priority in their lives.

Sexual health promotion and the development of culturally appropriate sexual health information and services are further hampered by a lack of good quality data regarding minority ethnic communities at both national and regional levels. The more detailed data collected in the April 2001 census will help, and the 2001 implementation of the Race Relations (Amendment) Act will require the development of specific duties for the National Health Service, including ethnic monitoring of all service delivery.

There are no comprehensive statistics on teenage births or abortions by ethnic group. Information is collected based on the mother's country of birth but often this does not identify women from minority ethnic communities who are born in England. Some health trusts do collect this data but not consistently. However, it is known that, although there is huge diversity within communities, young people from Bangladeshi and Pakistani communities are substantially more likely to be teenage parents than the national average, in part because of traditions of early marriage and childbirth.

Barriers to sexual health information and services

Young people from Indian, Pakistani and Bangladeshi communities may face barriers to obtaining good sexual health information, support and services both because of the cultural and religious traditions within their communities and due to insufficient targeting or insensitive responses from service providers.

Given the culture of silence it may be difficult for young people to develop knowledge around sexual health in a confident and questioning manner. Some may not have had the opportunity to develop negotiation and assertion skills, compounded, for a minority, through withdrawal from school-based sex and relationships education classes based on parental perceptions that the content may not be culturally and religiously appropriate.

Even among parents who are otherwise willing to talk to their children, there may be anxiety and a lack of confidence: 'I know it is important for me to talk about these things but I am so embarrassed. No one spoke to me about sex when I was younger. I just don't know where to start or what to say'(Indian parent).

Many young people from Indian, Pakistani and Bangladeshi communities therefore have to rely on their peers, the media and siblings for information about sexual health issues. Whilst some of the information they access may be accurate, much of it may be misinterpreted, and reinforces existing myths and stereotypes.

These issues may be compounded by poor service responses, which make young people from these communities feel even more isolated through the perception that no one understands them or the cultural context within which they are living. For example, some service providers express fear and anxiety about addressing sexual health issues with young people from these communities, as it requires them to challenge taboos in ways that they feel might inadvertently offend the communities that they wish to work with. However, there are ways of engaging positively with these communities and developing culturally and linguistically appropriate service provision.

Moreover, even where appropriate services have been developed, young people may not always be aware of what is available to them locally, or the fact that these are free of charge and not necessarily linked to their GP. The issue of confidentiality in terms of service use is of heightened significance for these young people because of the taboo nature of sexuality and potential consequences of sexual activity if found out. Linked to this is the issue of some young people being chaperoned to and from school or college, leaving little free time to access health information or services.

In relation to service provision specifically, young people from these communities highlight a number of key barriers, including:

- institutional and personal racism
- lack of knowledge and understanding of different moral value systems
- inappropriate and inaccessible locations

- concerns about confidentiality
- no relevant images or culturally appropriate sexual health messages.

Foundations of effective working
Providing a lead in national policy

Developments at a national policy level are now addressing many of the broad issues relating to the sexual health of black and minority ethnic young people. For example, The Social Exclusion Unit report on teenage pregnancy (1999) highlights the need for sexual health advice to be better tailored to help young people from black and minority ethnic communities. The National Strategy for Sexual Health and HIV also highlights the importance of developing appropriate service provision for these young people.

Working in partnership

At a local level, it is vital to consider community development and working in partnership with organizations so that young people from Indian, Pakistani and Bangladeshi communities can be empowered and enabled to make informed choices about maintaining and preserving their sexual health proactively rather than reactively during crises. Positive involvement with communities increases the likelihood of developing appropriate sexual health interventions. Box 8.1 describes an example of this type of work.

Many young people from Indian, Pakistani and Bangladeshi communities do not readily access mainstream or specific sexual health services, therefore partnerships with other organizations are essential. For example, this can be done by identifying appropriate schools, youth agencies and social services departments that can provide initial advice and information on sexual health, then facilitating referral to specialist agencies. If there is positive engagement with community-based organizations already working with these communities, information and advice can be provided in a much more appropriate way, making it more likely to have a positive impact.

By combining the skills of staff experienced in relating to these young people with the expertise of sexual health professionals, joint working can offer more of a one-stop service, and allows professionals themselves to learn new information and skills that they can then take back to their individual services. Sharing resources such as information, human or financial, can also facilitate efficient working, extending service provision beyond what might be achieved independently.

In considering joint working in this area, many of the general principles of effective partnerships apply. In particular it is important that there is a shared understanding of how work will be undertaken in a respectful and anti-discriminatory way.

Box 8.1 Case study: Guidelines for service providers on sexual health work with Hindu communities

In 1999, community work was undertaken with Hindu communities living in Birmingham to facilitate the production of these guidelines. The same process was also undertaken with local Sikh and Muslim communities around the production of sexual health guidelines for service providers working with these particular communities. This lengthy process was initiated by the Health Promotion Service of Birmingham NHS Community Health Trust.

The work involved the active participation of local communities across all sections, and ensured that there was a balanced representation of men, women and young people from each of the local communities that were being targeted as part of this work. Single and mixed gender workshops were organized so that people could share what they considered was essential to include in the guidelines for local service providers. Young people were engaged in the discussion of potentially contentious sexual health issues by using drama. This was also used as a technique for engaging adult audiences in discussions about culturally taboo issues such as HIV infection.

Contrary to popular belief, the parents and carers involved in this process were fully aware of the premarital sexual behaviour of the young men from their communities, although this was not openly discussed.

Throughout the development of the sexual health guidelines they highlighted the importance of the young men needing to 'protect' themselves by practising safer sex when visiting sex workers. They also acknowledged that sexuality was a difficult issue for them to address, but readily accepted that there were young men and women within their communities who may prefer to engage in same-gender sexual relationships. This clearly highlighted some of the tensions which existed within these communities where remaining unmarried would be perceived as a cultural aberration.

Developing effective services

Key questions

The following questions may help in identifying what services are already available to promote the sexual health of young people from Indian, Pakistani and Bangladeshi communities and how these can be enhanced:

- What provision is there for young people from these communities in your locality and who is working with and representing these young people?

- What partnerships and collaborative working arrangements exist around work with young people from these communities? Could these also integrate issues around sexual health advice?
- What examples of best practice in contraceptive and sexual health services for these young people have already been developed in your locality? Are they transferable? What lessons have been learnt?
- What support exists in your locality for teenage parents from Indian, Pakistani and Bangladeshi communities?
- What work is currently being developed with the parents and carers, since they are very important when it comes to positively endorsing and supporting work with these young people?
- Is there a programme of service development which actively involves young people from these communities in both policy and service provision issues?

Set-up issues

Staff training and development

Young people from Indian, Pakistani and Bangladeshi communities express concerns about their experiences of staff attitudes within sexual health services. Non-judgemental attitudes and clarity about what constitutes anti-discriminatory practice within each service provision agency need to be agreed and demonstrated by all staff including volunteers and interpreters.

This should be followed by ongoing support, training and adequate supervision to ensure that staff are confident to work with the range of diversity amongst young people from these communities.

Environmental issues

Services need to reflect the diversity across and within local communities. Consideration needs to be paid to the décor, including culturally and linguistically appropriate posters, leaflets, magazines and newspapers. The use of culturally and linguistically appropriate radio and television programmes can also help to create a more informal and welcoming atmosphere. Above all, attention needs to be paid to the welcome extended to young people from these communities by the staff, to ensure that the atmosphere is conducive to their seeking help without fear, intimidation or worries about confidentiality.

Accessibility

The location of services is a prime concern. This needs to be balanced with ease of accessibility and anonymity, given the taboo nature of sex and sexuality for young Indian, Pakistani and Bangladeshi people. An example of service provision which ignored this cultural context was where a walk-in centre was located near to a taxi company that employed a significant proportion of drivers from local Indian and Pakistani communities; as a result, young people from these communities avoided the service due to concerns around confidentiality and not wishing to be seen entering the centre by other people from their communities.

Service opening hours also need to take account of the potential call of other cultural and religious duties on young people's availability: for example, prayer or language classes after school or at weekends.

Generic services where sexual health is one element of other activities can be a helpful way of providing safe access for these young people. In particular the school nurse may be a vital resource for young people from Indian, Pakistani and Bangladeshi communities who may not be able to access services easily outside the confines of the school environment.

Given the cultural sensitivity of sex and relationships and the differential power relationships that exist between genders in Indian, Pakistani and Bangladeshi communities, gender-specific sessions for young people may often be appropriate.

Publicity

Service providers can sometimes lack awareness of how to communicate about the services they offer in terms of sexual health using culturally appropriate language and terminology. Information, resources and general publicity materials may not be sufficiently tailored in this regard. This can be addressed through direct consultation with local communities, engaging the local media, parents/carers and young people themselves in preparing and promoting existing or planned services.

Monitoring and evaluation

As with any service, monitoring and evaluation help to track whether targeted resources and interventions are having an impact. Specific indicators of success with Indian, Pakistani and Bangladeshi communities might include an increase in the number of young people accessing services, an increase in staff confidence to meet the sexual health needs of young people from these communities, and improved engagement with local communities about service development. These in turn should have an impact on sexual health outcomes for these young people.

Conclusion

Sexual health work with young people from Indian, Pakistani and Bangladeshi communities is still evolving. Greater efforts to actively involve these young people in all aspects of service development, from policy through to frontline service provision, are likely to yield positive results. Sensitivity in terms of understanding the position of young people in these communities and the kinds of pressures and conflicts they may face is also vital. Work on both these fronts should result in more inclusive, appropriate and non-threatening approaches, both within the health service and in partnership with other sectors. While this is a real challenge for all parties involved – practitioners, service providers, policy makers, local communities and young people themselves – it is imperative if existing gaps and inadequacies are to be addressed. Significant improvement will take time, and some of the influencing cultural factors are deeply rooted and not easily changed. However service providers can go a long way by ensuring young people in these communities can access the information, skills and confidence to explore and protect their sexual health.

References

Department of Health (2001) *Better Prevention, Better Services, Better Sexual Health. The National Strategy for Sexual Health and HIV*. London: Department of Health.

Social Exclusion Unit (1999) *Teenage Pregnancy*. London: The Stationery Office.

Teenage Pregnancy Unit (2001) *Guidance for Developing Contraception and Sexual Health Advice Services to Reach Black and Minority Ethnic (BME) Young People*. London: Department of Health.

Useful resources and organizations for working with Indian, Pakistani and Bangladeshi young people

Resources

Birmingham Specialist NHS Community Trust (1999) *Guidelines for Service Providers Working with Hindu, Sikh and Muslim Communities*. Birmingham: Birmingham Specialist NHS Community Trust.

Blake, S. and Lawrence, P. (2003) *Optimus Management Briefing for Schools – Promoting Race Equality: Policy Into Practice*. London: Optimus.

House of Commons Health Committee (2002) *Sexual Health Third Report of Session 2002/2003* 1. London: HMSO.

Katrak, Z. and Blake, S. (2002) *Faith, Values and Sex and Relationships Education*. London: National Children's Bureau.

Katrak, Z. and Scott, I. (2002) *Diverse Communities: Identity and Teenage Pregnancy. A Resource for Practitioners*. London: Teenage Pregnancy Unit.

North West Lancashire Health Promotion Unit (1997) *Mazab and Sexuality – Faith and Sexuality – A Discussion Paper on Sexual Health for Health and Community Workers from Four Faith Perspectives*. North West Lancashire Health Promotion Unit.

Useful organizations

Black Health Agency
Zion Community Health and Resource Centre
339 Stretford Road

Hulme
Manchester M15 4ZY
Tel: 0161 226 9145
www.blackhealthagency.org.uk

Commission for Racial Equality
St. Dunstan's House
201–211 Borough High Street
London SEI IGZ
Tel: 020 7939 0000
www.cre.gov.uk

Institute for Race Relations
2–6 Leeke Street
London WCIX 9HS
Tel: 020 7837 0041/ 020 7833 2010
www.homebeats.co.uk

9 Sexuality and Learning Disability

SUSAN DOUGLAS-SCOTT

> **Key issues**
>
> - Free, informed choices about sexuality and sexual expression are basic rights for young people with learning difficulties. However, social and cultural factors create barriers to these rights being maintained.
> - Parental and professional concerns about consent and risk of sexual exploitation or abuse can lead to the sexuality of young people with learning difficulties being controlled by others.
> - A lack of understanding of social norms can result in young people with learning difficulties behaving inappropriately in public. This presents problems for them and for their supporters.

Overview

This chapter examines the complex issues raised for young people with learning difficulties, their parents, carers and support staff in relation to sex education, sexual health and sexuality. It argues that many of the problems that these groups face are often the result of specific cultural and societal barriers rather than intellectual impairment (Goble, 2002). If these barriers are acknowledged, it is then possible to identify potential solutions to assist people in understanding the issues on their own terms.

Introduction

This chapter talks about 'learning difficulties' in relation to the young people who are the focus of discussion. Selecting terminology in this area is difficult, in particular because of debates about who is included in a definition and what connotations arise from choosing one label over another. The term 'learning difficulties' came from within the disability movement as a term of self-empowerment, and is now widely used. It includes a wide range of people who have intellectual impairments (such as Down's syndrome), who find it difficult but not impossible to learn, and who rely on families, carers and services to help them make sense of daily tasks and social situations and to maximize their independence.

It is recognized that young people with learning difficulties grow up in many different circumstances that have implications for their health and wellbeing. For example, those who have learning difficulties and are looked after by local authorities may face multiple risks in relation to sexual health outcomes, such as those in relation to unplanned teenage pregnancy and in relation to exploitation. However, because of space limitations this chapter will focus more on general issues.

Following a description of some general issues for young people with learning difficulties and their families, the chapter focuses on issues relating to sexuality and sexual health. It examines the current response of disability services and health services and outlines what more is required to better enable young people with learning difficulties to express their sexuality in a healthy way.

Scale of the issue

Because of the different ways of labelling those with learning difficulties, it is difficult to provide exact figures on the number of young people who rely on support from those around them to understand and access information. Even within Learning Disability Services, teams of staff support people with very different needs. These range from complex support needs due to multiple sensory, physical impairment and intellectual impairments to mild learning difficulties.

The 1990 census suggests that overall around 7.3 per cent of the population are affected (British Council). Further data sources provide some idea of the scale of the issue in Scotland and England.

England

- Around 160,000 adults have severe/profound learning difficulties.
- Between 0.45 and 0.6 per cent of children (55,000 to 75,000) have moderate to severe learning difficulties.
- The number of people under the Learning Disability speciality in NHS hospitals and units in 1999 was over 7000.
- The number of residential care places for people with learning difficulties in 1999 was over 51,000.

(Source: www.doh.gov.uk/learningdisabilities/facts.htm)

Scotland

- An estimated 120,000 Scottish people have learning difficulties.
- 20 people in every 1000 have mild or moderate learning difficulties.

- 3–4 people in every 100 have severe learning difficulties with complex support needs.
- 4000 to 5000 young people under 16 need a lot of help with daily living; another 4000 to 5000 require a great deal of support.
- In September 1998, there were 8800 children with learning difficulties in mainstream school. Some 37,700 children have special education needs (5 per cent of all children).

(Sources: Scottish Executive, 2000; NCH Scotland, 2003)

General issues in addressing sexuality and sexual health needs

People with learning difficulties are inherently sexual, have the same range of sexual preferences and behaviours as non-disabled people (Brown, 1994), and have the same rights to free and safe sexual expression as anyone else. However, society does not easily view them as sexual beings, but rather sees them as needing to be protected from sexual information and relationships. Unlike non-disabled young people, people with learning difficulties are not encouraged to consider themselves as having a sexually active future, including reproduction and parenting (McCarthy and Thompson, 1993).

Disabled feminists have for over a decade expressed concern about sexual oppression and exclusion, suggesting that lack of willingness to accept or even acknowledge disabled people as sexual beings is a major barrier to independent living (Finger, 1991; Morris, 1991; Morris, 1993; Keith, 1994). Stereotyping (Shakespeare, 1994) and a lack of capacity to see people with learning difficulties as anything other than vulnerable people adds to the difficulties in providing appropriate support.

While on the one hand young disabled people are generally not seen as sexual, on the other hand, there is a myth that they are overly sexed and that information and discussion about sex only encourages them to be sexualized in their behaviour (Thompson et al., 1997). Yet some of the inappropriate behaviour that does occur often results from a lack of information, for example in relation to private and public touching and body exposure.

Gaining balanced and accurate information on sex education, sexual health and sexuality can be a minefield for all young people (Burtney, 2000; Wight et al., 2002). For young people with learning difficulties in particular, accurate, comprehensible information is often inadequately provided (Schwier and Hingsburger, 2000; McConkey and Ryan, 2001). Sexual images and information are widely available and convey confusing messages: on the one hand there is a clear message to wait until they are older before becoming sexually active; on the other they are bombarded with messages suggesting that sex is something everyone is engaging in.

Young people with learning difficulties face multiple challenges in relation to gaining balanced information and support, are much less likely to access sex and relationships education than their non-disabled peers (Hopkins, 2003), and are more likely to encounter barriers arising from a number of sources (Stewart and Ray, 2001). Yet their need for targeted sex and relationships education may be even greater because of the additional risks to personal safety and health that they may face. While it is not possible from the data available to outline the extent of health outcomes for people affected by learning difficulties, it seems fair to conclude that both men and women with learning difficulties are likely to experience poorer sexual health.

The challenge for everyone involved with a person with learning difficulties is to empower that individual to express his or her wishes and assist him or her to live an ordinary life in his or her chosen community setting (Snow, 1991). We need to expand definitions of 'intelligence' and 'social functioning' and, in relation to sexuality, recognize that people with learning difficulties have the same range of sexual drives, desires and needs as the rest of the population. It then becomes necessary to identify the range of support needs around sex education, sexuality and sexual health that have to be addressed if people with learning difficulties are to become sexually empowered.

Concerns about exploitation and abuse

As well as supporting their rights to fulfilling and safe sexual expression, a key reason to educate young people with learning difficulties about their bodies and sex is to inform them about the potential for sexual abuse. People with learning difficulties are more at risk of sexual abuse than their non-disabled peers (Johnson et al., 2002), not least because abusers are often concerned to keep their behaviours secret and may therefore target those who cannot fully understand or use language. Even within outwardly consensual relationships, McCarthy (1999) found that there were often high levels of coercion in relation to sexual activity by male partners, which the women with learning difficulties accepted as matter of fact.

A common response of parents and professionals to limit risks of abuse is to try to tightly control the behaviour and personal space of young people with learning difficulties. However, for many of these young people, being equipped with the information to identify what is sexually inappropriate and, with the knowledge that they have, the right to refuse unwarranted sexual advances is preferable to overly strict controls. Knowing more about the biology of sex, the concept of consensual relationships and the facts of sexual abuse, and being more assertive about expressing what they will accept in relation to relationships and sex should also enable them to be safer, both in terms of sexual health and in terms of risks of exploitation and abuse.

Providing these young people with the right words and concepts about healthy sexuality should also enable them to express concerns about abusive situations they may have been in. This should allow for quicker detection and response. Similarly, parents and professionals need to improve their ability to spot behaviour that might be indicative of abuse having occurred. For example, whereas inappropriate sexual behaviour by non-disabled young people may lead to suspicions that they have experienced abuse, because young people with learning difficulties are not perceived as being physically attractive such behaviours are sometimes attributed to their impairment rather than to underlying causes (Shakespeare, 1996).

Protecting young disabled people from exploitation and abuse is undoubtedly difficult. However, acknowledging their sexuality, providing them with the language with which to talk about sex, and giving them privacy to develop intimate relationships are not necessarily at odds with this, and are vital in terms of their individual human rights to free and safe sexual expression. Currently the response of many parents and professionals to the sexual health needs of these young people takes insufficient account of these issues.

Legal and policy framework

So how do we get a balance between the rights of the young person with learning difficulties to know about sex and sexuality, and the need to protect vulnerable young people from potential abuse?

There are various national and international legislation and policy guidance designed to protect young people's right to information, education and support, and to protect them from abuse. These provide guidance on what we can and cannot do sexually, and they define people with learning difficulties, their rights and their ability to consent. Relevant issues are covered in legislation relating to a wide range of areas, including education, children and young people, human rights and mental health. Although specific laws and policies differ, the emphasis with respect to people with learning difficulties is similar across the UK, and this section reflects mainly the overall ethos.

The Human Rights Act 1998 was implemented in the UK in October 2000. It brought a number of human rights issues to the fore and, in law, supports other pieces of legislation to ensure that people are treated fairly. No one is exempt and so it applies equally to people with learning difficulties. The Act covers issues relating to privacy (Article 8), the right to marry and have children (Article 12) and freedom from discrimination (Article 14). It also covers issues relating to sexual rights. The recent introduction of the Act means that much remains untested in practice and it remains unclear how it will make a real difference for people with learning difficulties.

In relation to the legality versus illegality of sexual intercourse for people with learning difficulties, the basis of defining this relates only to women and to men who have sex with men. For example:

- If a man were married to a woman with learning difficulties, then sex is legitimate.
- For unmarried women it depends on an assessment on the level of the woman's impairment of intelligence and social functioning.

(Sources: Mental Health Act 1983 in England and Wales; Mental Health (Scotland) Act 1984; McKay, 1991)

Under this definition, the question of consent is irrelevant. Therefore if a woman were assessed as 'having arrested or incomplete development of mind, including significant impairment of intelligence and social functioning' then it would be illegal for a man to have sex with her. If she were deemed 'capable' then it would not be an offence. With regard to same-sex relationships, the Criminal Justice Act 1980, section 80 makes 'homosexual acts' with a man with learning difficulties an offence if he cannot consent. As with vulnerable women, an assessment of capacity would be needed.

Capacity is considered as something that can be developed, and its centrality as an issue with respect to the legality of sexual contact illustrates why it is vital that those supporting people with learning difficulties help them to develop ways to express their wishes, desires and needs regarding sex and relationships.

In relation to people receiving care, the law focuses on issues of abuse rather than on ordinary development and expression of love, sexuality and sexual behaviour. For example, certain aspects of mental health legislation were designed to protect 'mentally disordered' people – including those with learning difficulties and mental health problems – from abuse by authority figures. In hospitals and nursing homes it is an offence for male staff to have sex with a woman or to engage in 'homosexual acts' with a man receiving treatment or support. Here the degree of learning impairment is irrelevant. The law is less clear about a female member of staff having sexual relations with a male service user. However, the duty of care would extend this to protect vulnerable men.

With regard to breaches of the law by people with learning difficulties, one of the key concerns is masturbation in public. This is an offence, and individuals with learning difficulties may need support to learn about the difference between public and private behaviour and about what is appropriate in which situations.

Those working to support young people with learning difficulties need to be aware of the legal and policy frameworks within which they should be operating. This includes the major policy and legislative frameworks outlined and also local education, social services and care commission policies. Specific organizations also need to ensure that staff are assisted and protected by relevant internal policies, and that staff training in relation to sexual health issues covers these (Johnson *et al.*, 2002).

Issues for parents and carers

Many of the issues raised above are challenging for parents and carers in relation to supporting the sexuality and sexual health of children with learning difficulties. Barriers to their providing adequate support include fear, embarrassment, not understanding the issues themselves, not having the right language to talk about sex, and not seeing sexual behaviour as legitimate for their children.

Despite the widespread presentation of sexual issues in society, parents and carers still have a key role in talking to their children about sex. Yet adults often find it difficult to talk about sex, particularly with young people. Many adults have not had adequate sex education at school and as a result feel lost when talking to their children, particularly those children with additional learning difficulties. Not having the right information and language with which to talk about sex can be a major barrier, and may mean that discussion is avoided entirely or that innuendo and inference are used, which only further confuses people with learning difficulties.

As discussed, parents and carers often have concerns about their child's capacity to deal with adult relationships and may view even older children as eternally 'infantile'. The controls on behaviour that they often impose as a result can mean little or no opportunity for privacy, particularly during the development of a relationship. Heyman and Huckle (1995) suggest that this creates delayed sexual development, not because of cognitive impairment but rather as a result of restricted learning opportunities.

Parents may also wish their children to share their perspectives on sex and relationships, particularly those that relate to religious beliefs. However, young people should be encouraged to make up their own mind and learn the importance of this as a life skill.

It is essential that parents are supported in understanding that if information about sex is not provided, their children will still have sexual desires and may still engage in sexual behaviour (Brown, 1994) and, crucially, that they have a right to this. Ignoring these needs may lead to confusion, frustration and challenging behaviour (Moore, 1991) and is likely to perpetuate some of the problems faced by young people with learning difficulties (Hopkins, 2003).

The role of teachers and support staff in sex and relationships education

Teachers and support staff working with young people with learning difficulties face similar issues to parents, with little specific training in how to communicate effectively with these young people about sex and relationships.

Young people with learning difficulties are supported in a range of settings, and get their formal education either in mainstream schools or in 'special' schools. Some of the latter are orientated around particular needs such as sensory impairment, while others accommodate young people with a range of impairments. This creates many challenges in terms of teaching styles and individual communication needs, and these challenges are amplified when it comes to communicating about sex and relationships.

The aim for all schools-based sex and relationships education (SRE) is to empower the young person to understand their bodies and their sexuality and the potential pleasures and risks of sexual relationships, and to make informed choices if and when they become sexually active. There are additional difficulties for teachers in communicating with young people with learning difficulties. This may be especially the case for those educated in mainstream schools, where sex education materials used and teaching methods may be less appropriate, and where lack of awareness can result in assimilation rather than true integration (White, 1998; Bisazza, 1999; Evans, 2002). Teachers themselves identify concerns, particularly where they have not had access to training in this area (Wight et al., 2002; Stewart, 2001).

The content of SRE for this group should not be any different from that of mainstream teaching, as everyone needs to know the same range of information about bodies, puberty, relationships, sex and sexuality (Eales and Watson, 1994). It is the approach that is taken in relation to the individual's cognitive and other impairments that is the key. Special schools are at risk of not fully addressing SRE (Stewart and Ray, 2001), finding it too challenging, and are likely to focus on personal and social development issues and risk management instead.

An assumption of heterosexuality dominates all SRE, and for young people with learning difficulties in particular this issue may be inadequately or not at all addressed. This may be due to social pressure, moral positions (Lawrence and Swain, 1993), teacher discomfort at discussing non-heterosexual sexual orientations (Brown, 1994; Buston and Hart, 2001) and the general expectation that these young people will not be sexual and certainly not be anything other than heterosexual in their orientation (Brown, 1994). However, young people with learning difficulties are just as likely to be lesbian, gay and bisexual (LGB) as any other young person, and such attitudes create major barriers, especially in relation to coming out for LGB people with learning difficulties. Staff influenced by these heterosexist views may need support themselves to understand same-sex issues before they can appropriately relay this information effectively to their pupils (McCarthy and Thompson, 1991).

Holistic SRE, covering all aspects of sex and sexuality, should also include information about same-sex relationships, provided in a way that meets individuals' cognitive abilities. Providing inadequate information may increase negative sexual health outcomes, for example in relation to young gay men with learning difficulties and HIV infection (Reed et al., 1992; Thompson, 1994; Mellan, 1995; Valios, 2002).

Underestimating the natural sexual desires of young people with learning difficulties, whatever their sexual orientation, and ignoring the potential behavioural responses to these, may mean that safer sex messages are overlooked. This may increase the risks to these young people from HIV and other sexually transmitted infections (Landman, 1994). In relation to young heterosexual women with learning difficulties there is the additional risk of experiencing unplanned pregnancy (Levy et al., 1992). The potential implications of unplanned pregnancy and early parenthood for these young women and for any children they have may be even more challenging than for young women in general.

Rather than ignoring sexuality or only responding when a sexual health crisis occurs, teachers and support staff need to be proactive in terms of SRE. Shakespeare (1996) criticizes this approach, suggesting that problems arise because disabled people's sexuality is ignored when it is not an issue, and is made too much of one if sexual behaviour manifests.

Barriers for services in providing sexual health support

Many health services and disability services and staff struggle to meet the sexual health needs of disabled people. Problems can arise where support services do not have adequate sex education and sexuality support policies in place, denying the rights of people who rely on such services to access information about sex and sexuality and to access appropriate sexual health services (Brown *et al.*, 2000). Even where general information about sex and sexuality is available from specialist sexual health services, this is not generally aimed at people who find complex concepts and the written word difficult to understand, and who may not have a level of independence to find appropriate information (Rushton, 1995).

Barriers include inaccessible information, comprehension barriers, staff with fears of how to 'deal' with disabled people and problems in accepting the sexuality of people with learning difficulties (Box 9.1). Services need to look at the needs of these young people and whether these are best served through mainstream provision or through specialist provision. On a practical level, services may need to consider how best to support people who may not be able to fit into short appointment slots, and who may be fearful of examination procedures unless they are explained in their own terms.

Box 9.1 Problems with mainstream sexual health services as identified by people with multiple impairments, including learning difficulties

- Expectations that disabled people with multiple impairments will not be sexual, resulting in little opportunity to explore sexuality or sexual behaviour, for example in relation to masturbation.
- Lack of privacy, especially for those dependent on 24-hour support, as staff 'police' relationships and access to sexual health services.
- Problems for professionals in understanding and communicating with those who may depend on a third party to interpret.
- Inflexible and poorly tailored information and support relevant to individual needs, not someone else's ideas of what is required.

Source: Designed to Involve, 2002

Conclusion

There is much to be done in acknowledging the sexual rights of young people with learning difficulties and in supporting them to express their sexuality in a safe way. Some of the changes required are at the level of social and cultural attitudes, others at the level of service delivery and support to parents. Key areas for attention are outlined below.

The language of the body

Young people with learning difficulties will understand formal and informal sex education better if they first have a grasp of the body and how it works. This can prove challenging for parents, particularly where things are repeated in public as the child learns what is acceptable and appropriate. Techniques such as Draw and Write may also be useful in communicating about issues relating to biology and the body (for example, Wetton and McCoy, 1998).

Accurate and consistent information

All young people need comprehensive information about sex and sexuality, and young people with learning difficulties need this to be provided in a way that is sensitive to their emotional and cognitive needs. This may mean providing information that is not simply in the written word and using more creative techniques to ensure that the information has been fully understood. In relation to sexual health, the right knowledge is required to dispel myths about getting pregnant, avoid unplanned pregnancy, avoid sexually transmitted infections, and access sexual health services.

It cannot be left to young people with learning difficulties to make sense of one of the most complex aspects of human relationships and behaviour. They are less likely to understand incidental learning and to see the relevance of social norms and need ongoing reinforcement from parents, carers and support staff. If windows of communication are established, these young people will slowly take in more information as their understanding grows.

Communication and negotiation skills

Skills relating to communicating and negotiating wishes and desires within relationships need to be developed. As with language, these skills need to be encouraged from an early age and built on over time. If this is done effectively, it can have a protective effect in relation to avoiding abuse. It can also facilitate young people with learning difficulties to:

- express pleasure and preference in sexual relationships
- delay having sex until they are ready

- consent to safer sex with their partner
- agree boundaries with their partner
- develop relationships that feel comfortable for them.

Young people with learning difficulties need opportunities to discuss emotions and feelings related to sex and sexuality and to develop positive attitudes to sex and their own sexuality. Parents in particular need to explore the best ways in which they can help their child to do this and seeking support from the wider family and appropriate professionals can be invaluable (Rushton, 1994; Schwier and Hingsburger, 2000). Resources designed to support parents at different stages are available (for example, Scott and Kerr-Edwards, 1999).

A holistic, lifelong approach

To ensure the fullest understanding for young people with learning support needs, sex education needs to be meaningful to boys as well as girls, young people from minority ethnic groups, young gay men, young bisexual people and young lesbians. For young LGB people with learning difficulties, learning about same-sex relationships and safer sex can have the twofold effect of increasing awareness of their sexuality and awareness of the risks of HIV and other sexually transmitted infections (Mellan, 1995; Valios, 2002).

Like all young people, those with learning difficulties will come back to questions about sex time and time again, with different needs at different stages in their life. There is therefore a need for a lifelong learning approach to sex education, taking account of the specific developmental and life courses and consequent needs (Stewart and Ray, 2001; Macaskill, 2003).

The central role of schools

In special schools, a more consistent whole school approach needs to be advocated, as well as more cooperation between schools and parents. This will mean that learning can happen across different settings and therefore be reinforced appropriately (Oliver et al., 1998). Without consistency, young people with learning difficulties will find it more difficult to understand where they fit in sexually and how to behave appropriately in different situations.

Teachers and staff addressing SRE for young people with learning difficulties should be teaching it within a context of confidence building, assertiveness skills acquisition and raising pupils' sense of self and others. By developing a programme that offers both formal and informal opportunities for learning, young people are more likely to develop the life skills they need to be confident adults in relation to their sexuality (Craft et al., 1996; Sex Education Forum, 1995; Brown et al., 2000).

Professional support and training

It is not only young people with disabilities and their parents that have learning needs in relation to sex and relationships. Support staff, teachers, health care professionals and policy makers with a role in promoting the sexual health of people with learning difficulties can benefit from training designed to build understanding and skills and challenge stereotypical views. Discussions about sexual discrimination need to be part of ongoing professional development within Learning Disability Services.

Balancing protection and rights

Young people with learning difficulties have the full range of human sexualities and sexual desires, with accompanying sex education and sexual health needs, and rights to express themselves sexually. However, they also have specific needs in relation to keeping safe. Striking a balance between these is challenging in a society that leans heavily towards seeing these young people as vulnerable and non-sexual. It requires better working between parents and professionals, in partnership with young people themselves and with the support of those who fully understand the complex issues. This should make it possible to better inform young people with learning difficulties and to help them, where they choose, to build strong, safe and fulfilling sexual relationships.

References

Bisazza, P. (1999) Special educational needs in East Surrey from a school doctor's point of view. *Journal of the Royal Society for the Promotion of Health* Mar 1999 **119**(1): 50–1.

British Council fact sheet http://www.britishcouncil.co.uk/diversity/disability_demo.htm

Brown, H. (1994) An ordinary sexual life?: A review of the normalisation principle as it applies to the sexual options of people with learning disabilities. *Disability and Society* **19**(2): 123–44.

Brown, H., Croft-White, C., Wilson, C. and Stein, J. (2000) *Taking the Initiative: Supporting the Sexual Rights of Disabled People*. London: Pavilion Publishing and JRF.

Buston, K. and Hart, G. (2001) Heterosexism and homophobia in Scottish school sex education: exploring the nature of the problem. *Journal of Adolescence* **24**(1), Feb: 95–109.

Burtney, E. (2000) *Evidence into Action Teenage Sexuality in Scotland*. Edinburgh: Health Education Board for Scotland.

Craft, A., Stewart, D., Mallet, A., Martin, D. and Tomlinson, S. (1996) Sex education for students with severe learning disabilities. *Health Education*, Nov 6: 11–18.

Designed to Involve (2002) *Sandyford Initiative Disability Access Audit*.

Eales, J. and Watson, J. (1994) *Health Education in Scottish Schools: Meeting Special Educational Needs*. Edinburgh: Scottish Office.

Evans, R. (2002) Ethnography of teacher training: mantras for those constructed as 'other'. *Disability and Society* 17(1): 35–48.

Finger, A. (1991) *Past Due: A Story of Disability, Pregnancy and Birth*. London: Women's Press.

Goble, C. (2002) Professional consciousness and conflict in advocacy, in B. Gray and R. Jackson (eds), *Advocacy and Learning Disability*. London: Jessica Kingsley.

Heyman, B. and Huckle, S. (1995) Sexuality as a perceived hazard in the lives of adults with learning difficulties. *Disability and Society* 10(2): 139–56.

Hopkins, G. (2003) Working progress: planning for sex. *Community Care*, 19 Dec–8 Jan: 42–3.

Johnson, K., Franley, P. and Harrison, L. (2002) Living safer sexual lives: research and action. *Tizard Learning Disability Review*, Jul: 4–9.

Keith, L. (1994) *Mustn't Grumble: Writing by Disabled Women*. London: Women's Press.

Landman, R. (1994) Making sex safer for people with learning disabilities. *Nursing Times*, 13 Jul: 35–7.

Lawrence, P. and Swain, J. (1993) Sex education programmes for students with severe learning difficulties in further education. *Disability and Society*, 8(4): 405–29.

Levy, S. R., Perhats, C. and Johnson, M. N. (1992) Risk for unintended pregnancy and childbearing among educable mentally handicapped adolescents. *Journal of School Health*, Apr, **62**(4): 151–3.

Macaskill, D. (2003) Living to learn, learning to live – learning difficulties and lifelong learning. *Tizard Learning Disability Review*, Jan: 29–33.

McCarthy, M. (1999) *Sexuality and Women with Learning Difficulties*. London: Jessica Kingsley.

McCarthy, M. and Thompson, D. (1991) The politics of sex education. Sexuality and long stay mental handicap hospitals. *Community Care*, Nov 21: 15–17.

McCarthy, M. and Thompson, D. (1993) Safer sex and people with learning disabilities. *Aids Health Promotion Exchange* 2: 11–13.

McConkey, R. and Ryan, D. (2001) Experiences of staff in dealing with client sexuality in services for teenagers and adults with intellectual disability. *Journal of Intellectual Disability Research*, Feb: 83–87.

Mellan, B. (1995) Sex on the line – not lives: educating people with learning difficulties about safe sex is no easy task. *Community Care*, 14–20 Sep: 30–1.

Moore, K. (1991) Confronting taboo: helping people with learning disabilities to understand their own sexuality. *Nursing Times*, Oct: 46–7.

Morris, J. (1991) *Pride Against Prejudice*. London: Women's Press.

Morris, J. (1993) Gender and disability, in J. Swain, V. Finkelstein, S. French and M. Oliver (eds), *Disabling Barriers – Enabling Environments*. London: Sage.

NCH Scotland (2003) *Factfile 2003: Facts and Figures about Scotland's Children*. London: NCH.

Oliver, D. P., Leeming, F. C. and O'Dwyer, W. (1998) Studying parental involvement in school-based sex education: lessons learned. *Family Planning Perspectives*, May/Jun **30**(3): 143–7.

Oliver, M. (1996) *Understanding Disability: From Theory to Practice.* Basingstoke: Macmillan.

Reed, N. A., Edwards, L. E. and Naughton, S. S. (1992) An AIDS prevention program for adolescents with special learning needs. *Journal of School Health,* May, **62**(5): 195–7.

Rushton, J. (1994) Learning together: research into the value of group work in teaching people with learning disabilities about sexuality. *Nursing Times,* 2 Mar: 44–6.

Rushton, J. (1995) Learning capers: people with learning disabilities need access to information on sexuality. *Nursing Times,* 19–25 Apr: 42–3.

Schwier, K. M. and Hingsburger, D. (2000) *Sexuality: Your Sons and Daughters With Intellectual Disabilities.* London: Jessica Kingsley.

Scott, L. and Kerr-Edwards, L. (1999) *Talking Together…About Growing Up. A Workbook for Parents of Children with Learning Disabilities.* London: FPA.

Scottish Executive (2000) *The Same as You?* Full report available on www.scotland.gov.uk/ldsr/

Sex Education Forum (1995) Developing sex education for pupils with learning difficulties. *Sex Education Matters,* Winter. London: National Children's Bureau.

Shakespeare, T. (1994) Cultural representations of disabled people: dustbins for disavowal? *Disability and Society* 9(3): 283–300.

Shakespeare, T. (1996) Power and prejudice: issues of gender, sexuality and disability, in L. Barton (ed.), *Disability and Society: Emerging Issues and Insights.* New York: Longman.

Snow, D. (1991) Teaching clients about sexuality: sex education for people with mental handicaps. *Nursing Times,* 22 May: 66–7.

Stewart, D. and Ray, C. (2001) Ensuring entitlement: sex and relationships education for disabled children. *Sex Education Matters,* Autumn. London: National Children's Bureau.

Stewart, S. (2001) *2001 A Sex Education Odyssey?* Conference Report. London: FPA.

Thompson, D. (1994) *Men with Learning Disabilities, Sex with Men in Public Toilets: Taking Responsibility.* British Sociological Association Conference paper.

Thompson, D., Clare, I. and Brown, H. (1997) Not such an 'ordinary' relationship: the role of women support staff in relation to men with learning disabilities who have difficult sexual behaviour. *Disability and Society,* **12**(4): 537–92.

Valios, N. (2002) Learning to love safely: gay people with learning difficulties have few outlets through which to explore their sexuality and little support from their carers, leaving many isolated or even in danger. *Community Care,* 28 Mar–3 Apr: 32–3.

Wetton, N. and McCoy, C. (1998) *Confidence to Learn: A Guide to Extending Health Education in the Primary School.* Edinburgh: Health Education Board for Scotland.

White, C. (1998) A battle to join mainstream [learning difficulties], *Community Care,* 28 May–3 Jun: 6–7.

Wight, D. and Buston, K. (2003) Meeting the needs but not changing the goals: evaluation of in-service teacher training for sex education. *Oxford Review of Education.*

Wight, D., Raab, G., Henderson, M., Abraham, C., Buston, K., Hart, G. and Scott, S. (2002) Limits of teacher delivered sex education: interim behavioural outcomes from a randomised trial. *British Medical Journal* **324**, 15 June: 1430–5.

Resources and organizations for working on issues relating to young people with learning difficulties

Ann Craft Trust: www.anncrafttrust.org

BILD *Your Good Health.* [12 illustrated booklets to inform people with a learning disability about health issues and explain how to get help for a variety of health issues. The booklets can be ordered separately. Price £5 and also available on tape.] http://www.bild.org.uk/publications/your_very_good_health_details.htm

Brown, H., Croft-White, C., Wilson, C. and Stein, J. (2000) *Taking the Initiative: Supporting the Sexual Rights of Disabled People.* London: Pavilion Publishing and JRF. [Provides an overview of issues facing disabled people in relation to sexuality and personal relationships, and of positive service initiatives designed to address them. It is intended for a wide audience and takes a disability right approach.]

FPA (2000) *Reach Out Training Pack: Personal Relationships, Sexuality and Needs of African and Asian Descent Learning Disabled People.* London: FPA. [Training pack for professionals and carers working with adults with learning difficulties and includes tried and tested exercises. Includes a comprehensive section on preparation and planning, and sample workshops, which can be used to plan training sessions.]

Gunn, M. J. (1996) *Sex and the Law: A Brief Guide for Staff Working with People with Learning Difficulties.* London: fpa. [Guide to the law in England and Wales. Topics include, sexual intercourse (age of consent, under-age sex, rape), sexual behaviour, marriage and divorce, sexual abuse, medical treatment, homosexuality, relationships between staff and carers.]

Jackson, E. and Jackson, N. (2000) *Helping People with a Learning Disability Explore Choice.* London: Jessica Kingsley.

Jackson, E. and Jackson, N. (2000) *Helping People with a Learning Disability Explore Relationships.* London: Jessica Kingsley.
[Two user-friendly, illustrated books aimed at people with learning difficulties who can use them alone or supported by a carer to explore a range of issues, including sexual feelings and romance. Follow the adventures of five friends who share a house together.]

McCarthy, M. and Thompson, D. (1998) *Sex and the 3 Rs: Rights, Responsibilities and Risks.* Pavilion, Brighton. [Contains not only ideas and materials for direct care staff but also suggestions for service response, acknowledging that other people often heavily influence the sexuality of people with learning difficulties. Topics include: intimate personal care, heterosexual, lesbian and gay sex, pornography, marriage and divorce, and contraception.]

McCormick, G. and Shelvin, M. (1997) *Exploring Sexuality and Disability 'Walk Your Talk'.* London: FPA. [Advanced training manual offering a range of structured exercises and activities to challenge discrimination against people with physical impairment and/or learning difficulties.]

McKay, C. (1991) *Sex, Laws and Red Tape: Scots Law, Personal Relationships and People with Learning Difficulties*. Glasgow: Enable (Scottish Society for the Mentally Handicapped). [Guide to the law as it relates to learning difficulties and sexuality in Scotland.]

Melburg, K. and Hingsburger, D. (2000) *Sexuality: Your Sons and Daughters with Intellectual Disabilities*. London: Jessica Kingsley. [Designed to help parents build their children's self-esteem (whether their children are prepubescent or already adults) and educate them about sexuality and safety. Explains what to teach, when to teach, and how to teach.]

Norah Fry Research Centre Research: www.bris.ac.uk/Depts/NorahFry/

Scott, L. and Kerr-Edwards, L. (1999) *Talking Together About...Growing Up. A Workbook for Parents of Children with Learning Disabilities*. London: FPA. [Illustrated workbook for parents and carers of children with learning difficulties. Contains exercises to help introduce topics such as puberty, body parts, public and private behaviour, keeping safe, growing up, feelings and relationships.]

10 Not Aliens or Rocket Science: Young Men and Sex and Relationships Work

SIMON BLAKE

> **Key issues**
>
> - It is essential to consider the social context of how boys learn to be men to realise the potential implications for sexual health and sexual health work.
> - There are many reasons for the way in which boys and young men react to and approach sexual health work; it is important to understand and factor in the contradiction between external behaviours and internal thoughts and feelings.
> - Practitioners must develop an understanding of gender socialization and use this understanding to inform practical strategies for addressing the sexual health of boys and young men.

Overview

This chapter identifies key issues regarding the sexual and emotional health of young men. It outlines what it means to be a man and the main influences on this before presenting guidelines for effective working.

Introduction

Sexual health is inherently connected to gender and sexuality. It is concerned not only with the physical (for example, how many young people have STIs each year) but also with the social/cultural (for example, how young people behave with each other and with the opposite gender; how they negotiate their sexual and relationship desires), and with the emotional (for example, how young men and women develop in their social context and how they feel about themselves).

The last 30 years have seen unprecedented changes in gender roles and significant shifts in the labour market, altering traditional expectations and opportunities and blurring the lines between what is considered typical or

155

acceptable for either gender. This changing broader environment helps to shape attitudes and behaviour, and may generate a range of competing or even conflicting pressures on young men and women and how they relate to each other. It is also a key factor in effectively addressing their information and support needs in relation to sexual health.

Previously, sexual health policy directed activity toward teenage pregnancy and directed attention to young women. However, more recent policy recognizes broader socioenvironmental factors on one level while supporting work to improve self-esteem of young women and reduce power imbalance within relationships (SEU, 1999). At the same time, there is an increasing emphasis on young men focusing on rights (to adequate sexual and emotional health promotion) and responsibilities (as friends, partners and potential fathers). The Social Exclusion Unit report on teenage pregnancy identified young men as *half of the problem and half of the solution* and set out a raft of action points regarding the needs of young men that have been translated into local action (SEU, 1999). Across the UK, it seems that policy makers and practitioners are now increasingly asking not 'how do we change young men?' but 'how do we help and support young men to develop positive self-esteem and emotional resourcefulness?'

Despite this shift, work with young men is still in its relative infancy. A recent review of national practice confirmed a lack of strong conceptual frameworks, little evaluation of what works, and short funding cycles leading to unsustainable projects (Lloyd, 2002). In addition, professionals themselves sometimes lack confidence about the best approach to sexual health issues with young men, which is less likely to be the case when working with young women. And focusing back on the broader context, for both young men and women external influences often militate against a constructive, positive approach. For example, media headlines and adult anxieties about feckless boys – their sexual behaviour, crime, educational underachievement, antisocial behaviour and disaffection – remain common and are often the focus of a moral panic, reflected in punitive policy interventions that are 'hard on crime' and that punish young fathers who 'run away' from their responsibilities.

Yet while it is true that some areas of young men's lives give cause for serious concern – for example, violence between men particularly after alcohol is rife (Biddulph and Blake, 2001) and suicide rates are rising (Lloyd, 2000) – there is much to be positive about and an increasing knowledge about how to tackle the problem areas as well as a commitment to do so. The remainder of this chapter will focus on young men, precisely because this work is underdeveloped and the potential for including young men in our sexual health work is great.

What does it mean to be a man? The 'real man trap'

Although there is heterogeneity within the group – for example, race, class, disability, sexual orientation, and so on, and also in attitudes and behaviour

– the general patterns of gender socialization and expectations for young men in terms of behaviour are similar in the UK and are significantly different from those for young women (Blake and Laxton, 1998). These patterns encourage stereotypical notions of acceptable attitudes and behaviour, and these can negatively impact on young men's ability to manage their sexual health, as they offer a particular version of themselves based on stereotypical notions of what it is like to be a 'real' man: the hard, macho, all knowing young man who does not talk about sex, relationships and feelings. This impacts on all aspects of sexual attitudes, beliefs and behaviour, creating what has been described as the 'real man trap' (Blake and Brown, 2004). Aspects of this are shown below.

Being perceived as feminine or gay

By a young age (six or seven) boys can eloquently describe the attributes that they should have: emphasizing fighting and playing football. They are also acutely aware of what they should not be, that is, not gay or feminine (Wild, 1997). Sexism and homophobia are common (Mac an Ghaill, 1994; Mason and Palmer, 1996) and are often used as a means of proving their own masculinity (Holland *et al.*, 1993).

Not knowing enough, not being good enough

One of the dominant messages is that young men must know everything and must be the best. In this context, it may be better for them to drop out themselves rather than try their best and fail. This has implications for their commitment to education and how they look after their health (Phillips, 1993).

An example of worries based on not being good enough is in the use of condoms. It is often assumed that young men do not use condoms simply because they do not want to. This can be the case but there are also many young men who say that they would like to use condoms but are worried about a range of potential 'costs' such as embarrassment – 'will I lose my erection', 'what if I cannot put it on?' (Forrest, 1998).

Asking for help

The average young man is unlikely to ask for help and support (Springall, 1997). Instead he will try to manage on his own. This leaves many young men feeling anxious and worried, with clear implications for their health. A report from the Samaritans (Katz *et al.*, 1999) suggests that young men will contact them when they are absolutely desperate about emotional issues. There is a similar pattern with physical health; young men often access sexual health services at a chronic stage rather than as a form of prevention. Increasing efforts to encourage young men to use services as a result of the English

Teenage Pregnancy Strategy appears to be reaping rewards, with anecdotal evidence suggesting that some services are seeing increasing numbers of males attending.

Emotional responses

Boys and young men are socialized to hide emotional responses that might be considered more 'feminine', for example, 'big boys don't cry'. The pressure not to show emotional weakness in the form of fear or affection can be damaging in the context of relationships. Evidence suggests that men are worse at recovering from relationship breakdowns and divorce, and tend to drink more, have more time off work and suffer more depression. At the extreme, domestic violence may be partly a result of underdeveloped abilities to harness their emotions and thinking skills together to guide their behaviour positively.

How boys learn about sex and sexuality

The process of learning to be a 'real' man and the belief that 'boys will be boys' no matter what, sets in from an early age. What boys learn not only has an impact on how they develop as young men but also on how they learn about sex, sexuality and relationships.

Family talk

In the family sons often miss out on conversations about sex and sexuality. Whereas the onset of menstruation provides a starting point for conversations with girls, there does not appear to be an equivalent milestone for boys. The general silence of fathers on emotional and sexual issues provides a strong message that men are not supposed to talk about sex and sexuality (Biddulph and Blake, 2001). Many now grow up without the consistent presence of a father in the home from whom to seek information and advice.

If anyone does talk to them about sex and sexuality it is often female carers who, as they themselves confirm, often do not know enough about the stages of male pubertal and sexual development and the feelings that go with these (Sex Education Forum, 1997). What boys would really appreciate is somebody who is able to talk casually, openly and honestly about puberty, sex and relationships. Issues such as shaving, the voice breaking and 'uncontrollable' erections all need to be addressed without embarrassment or embarrassing them (Blake and Brown, 2004).

If sex is discussed in the family it will often be with a macho focus with an emphasis on being 'careful'. Young men are expected to be heterosexual (APPGA, 1998) and to want sex all of the time (Davidson, 1997). This is in striking contrast to how discussion about sex is often handled with girls, focusing on encouraging them not to have sex.

Friends

Young men often turn to their same-sex friends for advice about sex and sexuality, especially where information from other sources is lacking. While it is natural to seek information from peers, who can be a valuable source of mutual support, the problem is that much of what is provided in this environment is misinformation that can in turn put pressure on young men to behave in certain prescribed ways. In the male peer group, expectations about sex are high: everyone is expected to know all about it and certainly to want it all of the time (Lenderyou and Ray, 1997). Heterosexuality is presumed and behaviour that is regarded as in any way 'womanly' is strongly rejected (Holland *et al.*, 1993). Homophobia is rife and young men who are perceived to be gay are often subject to bullying (Springham, 1996).

Misleading, inaccurate information and inflated accounts of sexual prowess push a certain notion of what a 'real man' is (Lenderyou and Ray, 1997). This notion prevails despite the fact that many young men know that they themselves lie and suspect that this is also the case for others in the group. The need to lie to each other about performance is paramount and there is little room for expression of feelings, and certainly not for serious conversations to answer questions, address doubts and calm worries.

School

School offers informal messages about acceptable gender roles and patterns of behaviour as well as formal sex and relationships education (SRE). Boys are quickly exposed to messages about the types of subjects and sports they should be interested in and the way they should interact with others; generally reinforcing the macho expectations built up since childhood. Through engagement with teachers, and same or opposite sex peers, boys and young men continue to learn acceptable masculine behaviours (Mac an Ghaill, 1994).

In formal SRE, the emphasis on reproduction and biology can leave young men uninterested and reinforces the idea that sexual health, including relationships and emotions associated with sex, is women's business. This is a wasted opportunity since many young men report wanting more opportunities to explore what it is like to be a man in a non-threatening way (Davidson, 2003).

The media

Much of the modern media, and in particular specialist men's magazines, has an overtly sexual flavour. Although many broader social changes in terms of gender roles are reflected in magazine content, women are often still presented in a passive way, reinforcing the notion both that women are there to perform a certain role in relation to men and that men should regard them thus.

The increasing number of men's health and fitness magazines are almost exclusively heterosexual in focus (although there is a fast growing stable of magazines for gay men), with an emphasis on getting a great body and on improving sexual techniques, reinforcing stereotypical attitudes about male physical and sexual prowess. At the same time as traditional male roles are being endorsed, other images and expectations are emerging, bringing new and sometimes contradictory pressures. For example, there is a growing emphasis on grooming and 'finer' aspects of physical appearance, with skin and beauty products being heavily marketed.

Pornography

Another key influence is pornography. Although there may be other motivations for seeking out pornography, one drive may be curiosity arising when questions and issues are inadequately addressed elsewhere. So while young men are often criticized for using pornography because it denigrates women, it may sometimes be the only sure place they can go to find out how to do it. But while pornography certainly illustrates some of the mechanics of sex, it does so in a way that further reinforces traditional power relations in sexual activity, and in a way that pays scant regard to emotional or relationship dimensions. In addition, it may give rise to worry and concern and may promote risky behaviour. The sexual performance portrayed is often 'super-human' and contraceptive use is rarely negotiated. Young men attending a Brook Clinic have presented a whole range of concerns as a result of watching pornographic movies, including the amount of semen they ejaculate and how to 'make a woman scream' (Falola, 2000).

Sexual health work with young men

The range of ways that boys and young men learn about gender, sex and sexuality demonstrates how improving their sexual and emotional health transcends the traditional boundaries of health services. It requires a joined-up approach that enables young men to develop beyond pressures of 'performing' masculinity. It also means taking a more holistic and gender specific approach. In addition to providing information about puberty, how to protect against pregnancy and STIs, and where to access help and advice, there is a developing consensus that work with boys and young men should:

- Explore and clarify positive values such as respect for self and others, taking responsibility, and challenge gender norms and expectations.
- Develop and practise emotional and social skills such as assertiveness, negotiation, compromise, accessing help and saying 'I don't know' or 'I feel scared, please can you help me.'
- Ensure effective provision of sexual health services that are relevant and accessible to young men and increase the numbers of young men accessing services.

Effective working involves a range of well-established methods including the participation of young men and partnership working across professions, between statutory and non-statutory agencies and importantly with parents and carers. In addition to sharing resources and skills, partnerships have the potential to enable a limited supply of men working in this and related fields to be utilized effectively and offer positive role models. A clear policy framework will enable partners to feel confident and clear about their boundaries and responsibilities.

Beyond this however, it is vital that work is undertaken sensitively, taking into account different cultural and social backgrounds and helping to build self-esteem. This notion of developing self-esteem is vital, as young men need to be emotionally competent and value themselves in order to be able to look after their sexual health. However, while low self-esteem can be damaging to sexual health – making young men vulnerable to pressures from others and less able successfully to negotiate healthy sexual relationships – it is important to recognize that high self-esteem can also be damaging (Emler, 2001) and can lead to greater risk taking and feelings of invincibility. It is therefore important that positive self-esteem is developed in conjunction with a realistic assessment of risk.

Key to building self-esteem is an understanding that young men will often behave differently from expected and that often there is dissonance between behaviour and beliefs/feelings. For example, some practitioners say that sometimes when young men are at their most boisterous they feel most unconfident, scared and anxious. If the surface is scratched a different version of young men will be seen: a version rife with vulnerability, insecurity and indeed a desire to talk, to discuss and make sense of the world (Frosh *et al.*, 2001). An understanding of this double world, the external (that is, that which we see) and the internal (that is, the hidden anxieties and doubts) lies at the heart of any effective approaches to working with boys and young men. Key to success is finding ways to work with the internal and the external in safe and creative ways (Blake and Brown, 2004).

Guidelines for work with young men

Through recognizing the different perspectives outlined in Box 10.1 it is possible to understand the impact of gender conditioning upon young men's behaviour, and use this understanding to develop effective sexual health work. The following presents some learning points to consider when working with young men.

When carrying out group work with boys and young men, **start young**. SRE needs to start early to help boys think and learn about the different messages and stereotypes before they develop.

Involve young men and ask for their views and ideas and use these to

Box 10.1 Examples of common situations in SRE and services illustrating the gap between practitioners' and young men's perspectives

The following offers four common situations in sex and relationships education (SRE) and sexual health service provision and helps illustrate the gap between the practitioner's and young men's perspectives. Each situation is followed by a short commentary from the perspective of a young man and a relevant practitioner. When reading the practitioner and young man's perspective, consider the likely impact on a) how the practitioner will respond to the young men and what messages this offers and b) whether the young men will have gained relevant education and support.

Example 1

A group of young men are playing around in an SRE class about reproduction. They do not appear to be paying attention and are trying to distract the young women.

Practitioner's perspective

They are messing around as normal, they are not interested in sex and relationships education and clearly think that they know everything. Poor girls, they seem really interested as well.

Young man's perspective

This is really boring and a bit embarrassing. It is not relevant to us because it is all about the female reproductive bits. Why can't we do something a bit more interesting? If we tease the girls that will distract the teacher from this and she won't try to show us up again by asking us stupid questions. It's almost the end of the lesson.

Example 2

An SRE class focusing on condom use and a group of young men are saying that they would never use condoms because they don't feel right.

Practitioner's perspective

They don't want to use them because they are irresponsible and they don't care about their partners. They are stupid really because there are so many infections around. Oh well, if they will be stupid that's up to them.

Young man's perspective

I want to use one but I am worried that I might lose my erection. Damn, I would be really embarrassed to talk about using a condom. What if I cannot put one on? I wish I could say that and maybe the teacher could help. I can't, everyone would laugh at me and think I am a right wimp.

Example 3

A group of five young men go to a sexual health service together for the first time. They are sitting in the waiting room being really noisy and flicking through the girls' magazines really quickly and laughing loudly.

Practitioner's perspective

They are being disruptive and trying to make me feel intimidated. The young women here must be feeling really nervous. I wish they weren't here. If they have to come at all they could come on their own.

Young man's perspective

This is really embarrassing – thank god my mates are here. I wonder what it will be like when I get in. Will the doctor be nice to me? The receptionist keeps staring at us, and I feel really uncomfortable. I hope they hurry up.

Example 4

A foster carer is attempting to talk about safer sex to a young man in her care. He is laughing one minute and hostile the next.

Practitioner's perspective

I wish he would listen and talk to me. I know he is having sex and I am afraid a sexually transmitted infection or pregnancy will complicate his life even more.

Young man's perspective

I don't need this. I know she is trying her best. I just can't talk about it. Life is too difficult and complicated.

improve the development of education as well as health services. If practitioners ask young men for their views and ideas it is more likely that the service will be relevant to them and meet their expressed needs, thus encouraging their increased engagement. Practitioners confirm that boys and young men really enjoy being asked about what they need to know and how they want to learn. They are often unused to being asked and therefore it is important to help them in the process and ask clear and specific questions. Equally they may present issues and ideas that at first seem unreasonable or challenging. This may be to test your ability to answer their questions, or in order to save face in front of their mates and appear to be knowledgeable.

Develop working agreements. These are normally referred to as ground rules but changing the name signifies a shift in power and offers the possibility for practitioners and young men to really develop a positive agreement as to how they will work together.

Develop **rituals** that help create confidence and safety. If boys and young men are familiar with the process they are more likely to participate fully in it.

Use **their energy** creatively by using physical icebreaker games and adapting traditional exercises, such as a values continuum and asking them to physically move along the continuum.

Use **distancing techniques** that enable boys and young men to gain the information that they need without exposing themselves. Using case studies and scenarios that involve people like them, without asking for their personal experiences, will help them to gain the information they need whilst maintaining their external mask. Role play and creative expression such as arts and drama allow their fantasy and intuition to kick into play, and can help release them from behaving in stereotypical gender roles.

The evidence base for SRE (Health Development Agency, 2003) stresses the importance of connecting to **community advisory and support services**. Arranging visits to the service, visits from services staff and running mock clinics can all build confidence in accessing these services (Thistle, 2003). It is important to remember that some of the most important questions that boys and young men may have are: Where is it? How do I get there? How long will it take? Will I have to give my name and address? Addressing these questions will increase the likelihood of young men accessing services. Before referring boys and young men, where possible check that it is 'boy friendly' and that a respectful service will be provided. The best and worst advertising for a service is word of mouth. If it is good people will shout about it. If it is bad they will shout louder!

Explicitly **target young men** in advertising sexual health services. Many young men will assume that the service is not for them unless they are explicitly told different. In Sheffield, a credit card-shaped advert explicitly states '*young men welcome*', '*young black people welcome*' '*young gay men welcome*'. This provides a clear message for different groups of young people.

Ensure that the **waiting room** is welcoming to young men. Review the waiting room and consider:

- Are there positive images of young men?
- Are there magazines for young men?
- Are there posters or leaflets that offer explicit negative messages about young men?

Build their **trust** in sexual health services by offering as quick and positive a service as possible. For example, initially it may be helpful to simply offer condoms without an extensive consultation. As they develop confidence they are more likely to engage in longer consultation and ask for the help and support they need. If they are required to undertake an extensive consultation on their first visit it may frighten them and mean they do not return.

A minority of boys and young men will not be in school, accessing youth clubs or attending sexual health services. **Outreach and detached youth work, including mobile buses,** which takes services to young men, provides a positive framework for engaging with young men about sexual health.

Conclusion

As this chapter describes, over recent years we have begun to see a shift in emphasis towards a more 'boy-centred' approach in national policy. There is a whole range of policy initiatives in England that support the needs of boys and young men, such as the Teenage Pregnancy Strategy and the Sexual Health and HIV Strategy. There are similar initiatives in Wales, Northern Ireland and Scotland, although under different names.

Underpinning all of these initiatives is the important belief that the views of children and young people must participate in decision making. A range of guidance and good practice documents now require government departments across the UK to develop plans for involving children and young people. At local and national levels structures are being developed to provide boys and girls with the opportunity to express their views and participate in the solutions. This process of engagement has provided vital opportunities for young men to be listened to and is clearly influencing policy decisions. Specific examples include an advisory group for the Quality Protects initiative, an advisory group for the Children and Young People's Unit and the Young People's Advisory Forum for the Teenage Pregnancy Strategy.

As all the evidence from practitioners and an ever increasing body of research suggests, we need to move beyond demonizing boys and young men, and learn not to be frightened or intimidated by them, but instead to value them, to learn from them and to enjoy them. It is too easy to demonize them and activities that they participate in such as football, and to make sweeping statements such as that men's friendships are not as strong as women's. It is arguably more challenging both personally and professionally to value them as individuals and to ensure that education explores their reality and works with them to clarify their own positive values and develop their skills.

There is a danger that working with boys and young men develops as a specialism, undermining the confidence of workers who are in contact with boys and young men on a day-to-day basis. Young men are not aliens, and this work is not rocket science. Instead workers need to use and adapt the skills and techniques that are already part of their repertoire, and use an understanding of masculinity to inform their work. We need to keep asking, 'What is in it for the boys?' Gender conditioning inextricably informs how boys and young men look after their sexual health. Messages about gender and sexuality are insidious in society. We need a positive sustained effort to 'update' and 'change' the culture in which we live. We all need to work together to challenge the messages and positively acknowledge, encourage and reward boys and young men who ask for the help and support they need, value diversity and support their emotional and social development.

Improving sexual health is about changing the way we view the world and what we expect for boys and girls. It is working in partnership across traditional boundaries, with children, young people and their families to carve out a different future where boys and girls, young men and young women can develop and grow with confidence and a positive vision for their futures.

References

All Parliamentary Group on AIDS (APPGA) (1998) *Report of Parliamentary Hearings on HIV and AIDS.*

Biddulph, M. and Blake, S. (2001) *Moving Goalposts: Setting a Training Agenda for Sexual Health Work with Boys and Young Men.* London: FPA.

Blake, S. (1999) *Consultations with Young Heterosexual Men to Inform the Development of a Mass Media Campaign.* Unpublished report. London: Health Education Authority.

Blake, S. and Brown, R. (2004) *Boys Own: Supporting Self-Esteem and Emotional Development in Boys and Young Men.* Sheffield: Centre for HIV and Sexual Health.

Blake, S. and Laxton, J. (1998) *STRIDES: A Practical Guide to Sex and Relationships Education with Boys and Young Men.* London: FPA.

Children and Young People's Unit (2001) *Learning to Listen: Core Principles for Involving Children and Young People.*

Davidson, N. (1997) *Boys Will Be Boys...? Sex Education and Young Men.* London: Working with Men.

Davidson, N. (2003) *Building Bridges: Young Men, Sex and Relationships,* education pack and game, Working with Men.

Department for Education and Employment (1999) *National Healthy School Standard (1999) Guidance.* London: Department for Education and Employment and Department of Health.

Department for Education and Employment (2000) *Sex and Relationship Education Guidance 0116/2000.* London: Department for Education and Employment.

Department for Education and Skills (2000) *Bullying: Don't Suffer in Silence.* London: Department for Education and Skills.

Department of Health (2001) *Sexual Health and HIV Strategy – A Consultation Document.* London: Department of Health.

Emler, N. (2001) *Self-Esteem: The Costs and Causes of Low Self-Worth,* York: Joseph Rowntree Foundation.

Falola, G. (2000) *What About the Boys?* Presentation given to Brook Conference, January 2000. London.

Forrest, S. (1998) *Giants and Cuties: Learning to Be a Man.* Paper presented to Let's Hear It for the Boys Conference. Abbey Centre, London.

Frosh, S., Phoenix, A. and Pattman, K. (2001) *Young Masculinities: Understanding Boys in Contemporary Society.* Basingstoke and New York: Palgrave Macmillan.

Health Development Agency (2003) *Teenage Pregnancy and Parenthood: A Review of Reviews.* London: Heath Development Agency.

Holland, J., Ramazanoglu, C. and Sharpe, S. (1993) Wimp or gladiator – contradictions in acquiring masculine sexuality. WRAP/MRAP Paper 9. London: Tufnell Press.

Katz, A, Buchanan, A. and McCoy, A. (1999) *Young Men Speak Out: Some People Think Boys Don't Have Feelings.* London: Samaritans.

Lenderyou, G. and Ray, C. (eds) (1997) *Let's Hear It For The Boys; Supporting SRE for Boys and Young Men.* London: Sex Education Forum.

Lloyd, T. (2000) *Suicide – A Briefing.* Men's Health Forum.

Lloyd, T. (2002) *Boys and Young Men's Health: What Works?* London: Health Development Agency.

Mac an Ghaill, M. (1994) *The Making of Men: Masculinities, Sexualities and Schooling.* Buckingham: Open University Press.

Mason, A. and Palmer, A. (1996) *Queer Bashing. A National Survey of Hate Crimes against Lesbians and Gay Men.* London: Stonewall.

Office of National Statistics (2001) www.statistics.gov.uk

Phillips, A. (1993) *The Trouble with Boys: Parenting the Men of the Future.* London: Penguin.

Public Health Laboratory Service (2001) www.phls.org.uk

Qualifications and Curriculum Authority/Department for Education and Employment (1999) *National Curriculum Handbook for Primary Schools.*

Qualifications and Curriculum Authority/Department for Education and Employment (1999) *National Curriculum Handbook for Secondary Schools.*

Sex Education Forum. (1997) Supporting the needs of boys and young men in sex and relationships education. Forum Factsheet 11, London: Sex Education Forum.

Social Exclusion Unit (1999) *Teenage Pregnancy.* London: The Stationery Office.

Springall, L. (1997) Encouraging young men to access sexual health services, in G. Lenderyou and C. Ray (eds), *Let's Hear It for the Boys; Supporting SRE for Boys and Young Men.* London: Sex Education Forum.

Springham, N. (1996) *Telling Tales: An Exploratory Study of Young Gay Men's Experiences of Schooling in Tyneside.* Newcastle and Tyneside Health Promotion.

Teenage Pregnancy Unit (2001) *Improving Contraceptive and Sexual Health Services for Boys and Young Men.* London: Department of Health.

Thistle, S. (2003) *Secondary Schools and Sexual Health Services: Forging the Links.* London: Sex Education Forum.

Wild, G. (1997) Supporting sex and relationships education in the primary school, in G. Lenderyou and C. Ray (eds), *Let's Hear It for the Boys; Supporting SRE for Boys and Young Men.* London: Sex Education Forum.

Part Four

Learning About Sexuality

Introduction

There is wide acceptance that learning in general is a lifelong process, which is multifaceted in nature. This too is the case for sexuality, whereby we are continually facing new challenges to our existing knowledge, values and belief systems. This process of learning about sexuality is of particular relevance to young people as they come to terms with their own and others' sexuality, and it is an important time for supporting and encouraging young people to facilitate this process.

How young people learn

Undoubtedly young people learn about sexuality from a range of sources, the most commonly cited being school, parents, friends and the media (Todd *et al.*, 1999). It is often difficult though to attribute learning because often it is pervasive, as with parental influence, rather than overt, as with school-based sex education. Nonetheless, information will be assimilated at different times and in different ways across the lifespan.

One of the biggest challenges young people face is to decipher the mixed messages that are available to them. It has been argued that one of the reasons for high teenage pregnancy rates in this country is the confusion around sexuality: on one hand it is all around, yet on the other there is little open discussion or information available (SEU, 1999). In various parts of the UK there is concerted effort to start to introduce consistency of message across settings. For example, in Scotland the national health promotion agency (HEBS) devised a teacher-led sex education programme supported by a separate website for young people. The way which material is presented differs, but the health promotion messages remain constant: we need to be more open to discuss issues about sexuality and relationships.

However there are limits to the extent to which we can control the messages that are available. The media, which is often incorrectly thought of as one entity, has many facets through which young people learn about sex and sexuality. Some aspects of the media have taken on board sexual health issues: for example magazines aimed at young women will present information in a sophisticated manner and editors of a number of magazines have formed the Teenage Magazine Arbitration Panel (TMAP) to deal with complaints about sexual material. However, others use sex in a sensationalistic, tantalizing manner (Batchelor *et al.*, forthcoming). Is this wrong? These issues will be discussed in more detail in this section, but many would argue that the *raison d'être* of the media is to reflect back what young people want to hear and see, not to educate and lecture. The media is a commercial enterprise which sets out to make money rather than inform social behaviour.

Where should we focus?

In policy and practice terms, attention has been focused to a large extent on school-based sex education, as it is the most obvious formal setting for policy makers and practitioners to target. A captive audience is guaranteed and there is control about the way in which sexuality is presented and discussed. However, policy could be accused of over-emphasizing the importance of schools, given the limited time that can reasonably be devoted to this issue, especially in secondary schools where a traditional curriculum still dominates. One of the possible reasons work has not extended to include parents is the risk of being accused of fostering a 'nanny' state which could interfere with home life and parenting styles. However, there are a number of ways in which the importance of parents can be recognized and their information and support needs met. It is becoming increasingly recognized that the synergism of home/school partnerships has considerable potential for future development.

Work on parenting has already started and there are a number of government led initiatives. Within health, the national health promotion efforts in Scotland have invested in a series of parenting advertisements to support wider communication between parent and child.

This is indicative of the broader evidence, which supports generic work, in partnership with specific sexual health information to develop life skills that will facilitate better relationships. In addition there is recognition of the relationship between sexuality and other social and health issues in the lives of young people. For example there is increasing evidence to link alcohol and substance use with risky sexual behaviour.

The focus of this section

This section considers the four main sources of information for young people in the specific context of sexual health while exploring the broader influences of the media, parents, schools and friends. For example the way in which a child learns at school is dependent on the broader culture of the school and the extent to which the young person feels comfortable within the social environment of the school. The whole school approach is supportive of this notion, and it is being developed across the UK under various guises such as health promoting schools and community schools.

The challenge of each approach is explored in some detail: for example, peer education has many strengths but the underlying difficulty with trying to replicate a friendship network in an artificial way is not underestimated or fully understood. The importance of multifaceted learning is a further theme explored in the chapters to follow. For example, the influence in the home is tempered by interaction outside with friends, school and the media. Finally, the extent to which we can influence is highlighted, as in the media chapter (Chapter 14), which is a good example of the boundaries that are set, sometimes without our control.

References

Batchelor, S., Kitzinger, J. and Burtney, E. (forthcoming) *Representing Young People's Sexuality in the 'Youth' Media*. Health Education Research.

Social Exclusion Unit (1999) *Teenage Pregnancy*. London: The Stationery Office.

Todd, J., Currie, C. and Smith, R. (1999) *Health Behaviours of Scottish School-children, Technical Report 2: Sexual Health in the 1990s*. University of Edinburgh: Research Unit in Health and Behavioural Change.

11 Exploring the Role of Schools in Sexual Health Promotion

IAN YOUNG

Key issues

- SRE occurs best in a school environment where health is promoted in all aspects of school life.
- Schools need to move beyond an individualistic model to take full account of sociocultural aspects of sex and relationships.
- Realistic objectives should be set to reflect what could realistically be achieved through an educational approach and partnership working.

Overview

This chapter considers the strengths and weaknesses of schools as a setting for sexuality and relationships education (SRE). It outlines the background to SRE in the context of school-based health work and describes the general situation in the UK. A range of models and approaches to sex and relationships education are considered and key issues for developing a school policy in this area are highlighted.

Introduction

The potential for schools to contribute to health improvement became a reality in the late Victorian era (Young, 1993). The provision of a hot meal in the middle of the day was seen as a device to encourage attendance at school and also to improve the physical health and stature of young people; in time this became a state provision. Other health-related reforms followed, such as the development of a school medical service and the introduction of home economics as a subject.

The second half of the twentieth century saw considerable debate on the role of schools and education more generally. In 1976 Prime Minister James Callaghan's call for a 'great debate' on education produced a view that the curriculum in schools must reflect the needs of the nation rather than being

172

seen in more academic terms. Much of the discussion at that time related to producing young people who were able to serve the economic needs of the country. It has been suggested (Lewis, 1993) that once the curriculum started being used as a vehicle to respond to national needs, successive governments continued to use it to tackle 'crises' such as the HIV/AIDS epidemic.

Sex education in schools was not specifically on the agenda in the first half of the twentieth century. Indeed, in 1939 a government publication on health education in schools (National Board of Education, 1939) discussed the detailed provision of health education, including 'mothercraft', without a single reference to sex. But by the 1970s schools were seen as having a potential niche role for delivering sex education, especially since many parents were not adequately responding to the sexual education needs of their children.

Schools as a sexual health promotion setting

Schools never set out to provide the only response to SRE, and school-based SRE alone is unlikely to change behaviour, given the complex nature of sexuality and the range of influences as described in Chapter 2. However, as part of a multifaceted approach also involving parents and other significant influencers, schools have a number of strengths which can allow them to contribute to education for sexual health and relationships. These include:

- **Attendance at school:** most people attend schools between the ages of 5–16 years, for a total period of around 10,000 hours.
- **Trained educators:** while SRE is particularly sensitive, teachers are already equipped with core skills to facilitate learning.
- **Parental and young person support:** the majority of parents and young people support the role of schools in the delivery of sex education, although sometimes schools are used as an opt-out for parents.
- **Cohesive curriculum:** the school setting provides an opportunity for the development of a responsive SRE curriculum appropriate to the age and stage of pupils.
- **Links with other topics:** sex education helps to develop a set of transferable skills that are relevant to other aspects of life: for example, communication skills.

However, there are limitations to the input of schools in this area. First, schools may capture a large proportion of the population but there will always be those who miss out due to truancy, illness, religious background and so on. Second, schools can be seen as instruments of authority, which may be off-putting for some pupils and parents, and this links to the issue of confidentiality and disclosure. Third, schools have some difficulty with the sensitivity of the issues covered, particularly when teachers may not have received adequate training and support.

A further issue is the pressure on the curriculum with health promotion not being seen as the *raison d'être* of schools. Teachers and schools have their own targets and standards to meet and may have different priorities from other professionals with roles in sexual health promotion. This can create problems even for programmes that are explicitly designed to promote partnership between education and health. This is compounded by differing expectations regarding the successful outcomes of health promotion. For example, a programme may aim to delay or reduce sexual intercourse, which may lead to a reduction in teenage pregnancies or sexually transmitted infections. However, many in education feel this is not an appropriate way of measuring the success of their course given the influence of broader sociocultural factors. They believe that SRE should be measured against educational outcomes such as knowledge and understanding, and skills development of the students.

Partnerships between health and education are further complicated because in some respects the education sector talks a different language from health specialists. For example, the term 'curriculum' is conceptualized in some education reports in an all-encompassing sense to mean the totality of learning experiences that a school offers to young people. In health, the term is usually seen as the syllabus guidelines or the learning and teaching in the classroom. The broader influence of the school is encompassed within the concept of the whole school effect or the health promoting school. At the European conference 'Education and Health in Partnership' ten Dam explored the conference theme from an education perspective without having recourse to use the term health promotion once in her keynote presentation. She stated that the main reason for schools to be involved in health education was that it could contribute to the main task of education which she explained as identity development and learning to participate in society (ten Dam, 2002). In reality this example does not reflect a totally different vision from those working in health promotion. However the different use of language can obscure understanding in partnership working unless the partners explore each other's language and the concepts associated with it and come to some level of understanding.

Current provision of SRE

In the UK SRE is a component of the school curriculum; it can be located across the curriculum but tends to be prominent in personal and social education (PSE) (or equivalent) and in biology. Several policy and guidance documents form the basis of the curricula for SRE (Box 11.1). However, wide variation exists in the quality and approach to delivery across the four countries, across local authorities and between schools.

The objectives of a curriculum on SRE involve assumptions and judgments on what is important, what is acceptable and what is achievable. Traditional approaches in schools have often been based on the assumption that

Box 11.1 Key policies across the UK relating to sex education in schools

England

1988 Local Government Act Section 28

Local authorities prohibited from intentionally promoting homosexuality or publishing material with the intention of promoting homosexuality; and promoting the teaching in any maintained school of the acceptability of homosexuality as a pretended family relationship. This clause was subsequently repealed in 2003.

1996 Education Act

Set out mandatory SRE elements in National Curriculum Science Order, at the minimum in secondary school, to teach about STIs and HIV.

National Healthy School Standard (NHSS) DfEE 1999

Required local programmes to work with schools to offer challenge and support whilst contributing to whole school education and health improvement. SRE is one of the specific themes within the NHSS and the accompanying guidance to the Standard outlines the criteria for assessing school achievement in relation to SRE including the need for a specific policy, planned programmes, staff knowledge and confidence, and understanding of the role of schools in reducing teen pregnancies.

Teenage Pregnancy Strategy DoH 1999

Stated the need for improvement of SRE in schools at primary and secondary level. Provided guidance regarding the purpose and aim of SRE in schools.

Learning and Skills Act (2000)

Shifted responsibility for sex education from LEA to school governing body and head teacher.
   Stipulated importance of marriage to family life and stated that young people should be protected from inappropriate materials.

The National Curriculum DfEE 2000

Stated that schools should provide opportunity to learn and achieve and promote pupil development and prepare for life. SRE key strand of learning.

PHSE and Citizenship Guidance DfEE 2000

SRE highlighted as one aspect of holistic approach to meet four strands including good relationships and respect for difference, and healthy lifestyle.

Box 11.1 (continued)

NHSS Sex and relationship education guidance DfEE 2000

Guidance for local programme coordinators. At primary level guidance linked to age and stage of development but covering puberty, body knowledge, protection and confidence. At secondary level, beyond mandatory requirements of STI and HIV information, to prepare young people for adult life. Highlighted importance of communication with parents.

Northern Ireland

Guidance Circular 1987/45 DENI 1987

Established a framework for RSE recommending a written school policy on sex education endorsed by staff and governors and communicated to parents.

1989 Education Reform Order

Set out health education as a theme of the NI Curriculum.

HIV/AIDS strategy DHSS 1993

Highlighted the need for increased efforts in public education, alongside education programmes in schools and youth settings and support for those involved in providing sex education.

Production of guidance for teachers on health promoting schools NICC and HPANI 1994

Reinforced holistic approach to school health with aim of promoting lifestyles conducive to good health, including sexual health, supportive environment, and enablement of staff and pupils to take action for health community.

The Children (Northern Ireland) Order 1995

Stated statutory responsibility on Boards and Trusts to ensure the availability of a range of personal social services to support children in need.

Health and Wellbeing: Into the Next Millennium DHSS 1996

Stated that by 1998 schools should have developed and implemented a comprehensive health promotion programme in relation to sexual and reproductive health.

Circular 1999/10 Pastoral Care in Schools: Child Protection DENI 1999

Provided advice to schools and others on the responsibilities, in relation to child protection, which they have towards the welfare of the children and young people in their charge.

Box 11.1 (continued)

Teenage Pregnancy and Parenthood: Strategy and Action Plan 2002–2007 DHSSPS 2002

DE in partnership with Education and Library Boards, Health and Social Services Trusts and Health Promotion Agency will facilitate and support the implementation of the guidelines on RSE and progress will be assessed through the inspection of schools.

Guidance for primary and post primary schools on relationships and sexuality education CCEA 2001

Assistance for schools in developing a policy statement which reflects ethos of school and compliments existing school policy as well as in providing a programme of RSE appropriate to maturity and needs of pupils.

Development of regional sexual health strategy, DHSSPS 2003

Not yet publicly available.

Scotland

1986 Local Government Act Clause 2a

Like Section 28 in England but repealed in Scotland in 2000.

Personal Relationships and Developing Sexuality: A Staff Development Resource for Teachers, SOED 1994

Provided guidance to schools on approaching sex and relationships education.

Personal and Social Development: 5–14 National Guidelines, Scottish CCC 1995

Outlined support material taking the form of a workshop for teachers. It focuses on a whole school approach to personal and social development.

A Curriculum Framework for Children 3 to 5, Scottish CCC 1999

Described the scope of children's learning between the ages of three and five. It placed particular emphasis on their emotional, personal and social development.

Standards in Scotland's Schools etc Act 2000: Conduct of Sex Education in Scottish Schools

Complemented the Education Act 1980 and established the right of every child to have school education with an emphasis on the development of the individual child. It introduced rights for pupils to have views

Box 11.1 (continued)

known when planning and enabled ministers to issue guidance on conduct of sex education in schools.

Ethical Standards in Public Life Act (Scotland) 2000: Section 35: Conduct of Sex Education in Scottish Schools

This Act required that local authorities have regard for two principles in the performance of their functions relating principally to children. These principles are the value of stable family life in a child's development and the need to ensure content of instruction is appropriate with regard to age, understanding and stage of development.

Health Education 5–14: National Guidelines, LT Scotland, 2000

The revised guidelines provided an important curriculum context for sex education and highlight the close connection with personal and social development and the concept of the health promoting school. The guidelines are based on three interconnected strands – physical health, emotional health and social health.

Guide for Teachers and Managers: Health Education 5–14, LT Scotland 2000

This accompanies the 5–14 guidelines. It offers practical advice on a range of issues such as meeting pupils' needs and the health promoting school.

Report of the HIV Health Promotion Strategy Review Group, Department of Health

Highlighted the importance of SRE in prevention of HIV transmission and recommended that further advice and active encouragement be provided to education authorities by the Scottish Executive Education Department on how to deliver the curriculum objectives.

Report on the Working Group on Sex Education in Scottish Schools, SEED 2000

Following the announcement of intention to repeal Clause 2A (described above) this report set out the review of a package of safe-guards proposed by SE to address public concerns. Subsequently recommended a series of guidance publications to support schools, local authorities and parents.

Sex Education in Scottish Schools (McCabe committee), LT Scotland 2001

Series of publications aimed at local authorities, schools and parents to support the development of sex education in Scottish schools.

Box 11.1 (continued)

Enhancing Sexual Wellbeing in Scotland: A Sexual Health and Relationships Strategy, Department for Health and Community Care, 2003

The draft strategy considers the role of school-based sex education and in particular recommends that there should be a consistent approach to sex and relationships education across Scotland. This should be supported through multidisciplinary training and stronger links between education and services.

Wales

1988 Local Government Act Section 28

Details as for England, at time of press Section 28 being repealed in Wales.

Education Act 1996

Stated that pupils were to receive a broad balanced curriculum which promotes spiritual, moral, cultural, mental and physical development at school and of society and prepares pupils for adult life.

Building Excellent Schools Together Welsh Office 1997

Emphasized the importance of PSE as part of balanced holistic education, which equips pupils to be more healthy, effective and responsible in society.

2000 Learning and Skills Act

Requirement for National Assembly of Wales to issue guidance to ensure that when sex education is provided, schools must teach the nature of marriage and its importance to family life and the upbringing of children.

A Strategic Framework for Promoting Sexual Health in Wales 2000, National Assembly for Wales

Schools to ensure that all young people in Wales receive effective education about sex and relationships as part of their personal and social development.

Personal and Social Education Framework: Key Stages 1 to 4 in Wales, ACCAC 2000

Identified the sexual aspect as one which could be developed by schools through PSE, stating that 'as children and young people develop sexually

Box 11.1 (continued)

they need to understand bodily changes, manage sexual feelings and enjoy safe, responsible and happy relationships'.

Sex and Relationships Education in Schools, National Assembly for Wales 2000

Aimed to provide clarification on legal aspects, show how SRE should be taught in PSE framework, guide schools on sensitive issues, outline practical strategies and emphasize the importance of working in partnership with parents and the wider community.

an individual's health or ill health are to a large extent determined by individual lifestyle choices (Combes, 1989). This assumes that if young people develop appropriate knowledge, skills and attitudes then healthier choices and behaviours will result. However this model does not take full account of powerful sociocultural forces. As outlined in Chapter 2, the social environment, values and life expectations of young people are wider factors that any educational approach must recognize.

Current approaches are moving on from an individualistic model to a more social and holistic approach through the health promoting school concept (Scotland and Northern Ireland), the Welsh Network of Healthy Schools and the National Healthy School standard in England. The approaches have the potential to act as a unifying model for those involved in promoting health (Young and Williams, 1989), and may help raise the health profile and provide scope for schools to consider the formal as well as hidden curriculum.

They offer a flexible curriculum that recognizes young people's differing backgrounds, needs, conceptual frameworks and attitudes to schools, and uses these as a starting point for learning. This approach recognizes how the ethos of the whole school and issues beyond the curriculum may convey messages as powerful as any learning and teaching in the classroom. For example, if school toilets do not provide basics such as soap, towels, and bins for the disposal of sanitary wear, what does this say to young women having to cope with menstruation (Power, 1995)?

Sex education: approaches and delivery

It could be argued that there are two basic approaches to SRE from a health perspective: these could be stated as abstinence and comprehensive programmes. The basic theme of abstinence programmes, which are common in the USA (see Chapter 5), is that sex is only appropriate within marriage and that sex outside marriage will have negative emotional, physical and social consequences. This approach includes discussions about values and a focus on character building, and in some cases refusal skills.

There is little evidence to suggest that abstinence programmes have an effect on delaying sexual activity or reducing pregnancy. Kirby (1997) found no measurable impact on the initiation of sex, frequency of sex or the number of partners in a 12-month follow-up study of an abstinence programme.

Comprehensive SRE programmes, more common in the UK, aim to delay sexual activity until both partners are ready. They teach that sex is a natural, normal, healthy aspect of life and offer students the opportunity to explore and define their values and develop relationship and negotiation skills. This more pragmatic approach accepts that many teenagers will become sexually active and offers teaching about contraception and condom use (Collins *et al.*, 2002).

Comprehensive SRE programmes are associated with delay in first intercourse, and with increased condom and other contraceptive use at first and subsequent intercourse (Faculty of Public Health Medicine, 1995; CRD NHS, 1997). There is no evidence that comprehensive SRE leads to increased sexual activity or higher rates of pregnancy (CRD NHS, 1997; Wellings *et al.*, 1995; UNAIDS, 1997; Wight *et al.*, 2002). European evidence, particularly from the Netherlands and Scandinavia, indicates that good SRE can contribute to a reduction in teenage pregnancies, particularly when linked with access to services (Meyrick and Swann, 1998; Faculty of Public Health Medicine, 1995). An example of this approach is the SHARE[1] trial, which was evaluated between 1996 and 1999.

Kirby (2001) identifies key characteristics of effective sex and HIV education programmes, which he suggests should be grounded in theory. They cover aspects of the programme, for example, consistency and clarity of prevention message, accurate information, pupil involvement, skills based learning, recognition of social pressures, and aspects of delivery including the importance of a trained provider, adequate length of time and age appropriate teaching.

Delivering comprehensive SRE

SRE can be delivered by teachers, peers and/or outside agencies, often health professionals. Some models incorporate all three modes of delivery, others rely predominantly on one. Three major research projects in the UK have combined different delivery approaches (see Box 11.2).

Research comparing teacher-led versus peer-led SRE is limited; however findings from RIPPLE[2] indicate that a greater proportion of pupils taught by peers felt SRE was enjoyable, engaging and useful to them than those taught by teachers. Classes were better controlled when teacher-led.

Regardless of who delivers sex education, pupil satisfaction is higher when deliverers demonstrate high levels of expertise and motivation; a sensitive

Box 11.2 Synopsis of three major sex education programmes in the UK

SHARE (Sexual Health And RElationships – Safe, HAppy and REsponsible)

The aim of SHARE is to improve the quality of teenage sexual relationships, reduce unsafe sex and reduce unwanted pregnancies. The delivery of SHARE is through intensive teacher training to enable teachers to deliver active learning, using skills-based packs in intervention schools.

The design of the intervention took place from 1993–6 and the trial from 1996–2000. Both were located in the east of Scotland. SHARE continues to be delivered across a number of Scottish schools.

Evaluation to date

From 1993–4 a needs assessment and feasibility study was done and during 1994–6 the formative evaluation of the development of SHARE was carried out, with both of these pilots taking place in the same four schools. In 1996–2000 the randomized trial of SHARE took place, involving 25 schools with S3–S4 pupils and 5854 young people at follow-up. This was complemented by detailed process evaluation with pupils, teachers and senior management.

The period 2000–4 saw the follow-up of the trial to establish impact on terminations using NHS data.

Findings to date

Outcomes

Compared with conventional sex education, at age 16 SHARE:

- was evaluated more positively by both pupils and teachers
- increased practical sexual health knowledge
- reduced regret of first intercourse with most recent partner
- had no effect on age at first sex
- had no effect on condom or other contraceptive use.

The teacher training was evaluated extremely positively by teachers. It made them more confident and comfortable in delivering sex education, but did not lead them to prioritize skills development.

Processes

Faithful delivery of the programme was aided by intensive teacher train-ing, compatibility with existing PSE, and senior management support. It was hindered by competition for curriculum time, brevity of lessons,

Box 11.2 (continued)

low priority accorded to PSE by senior management, and teachers' limited experience in developing skills.

Most pupils reported being uncomfortable in sex education lessons, gender dynamics being particularly problematic. Their accounts suggest that their engagement in lessons depends on the teacher's role: maintaining discipline and preventing hurtful humour being crucial.

RIPPLE (Randomized Intervention of Pupil Peer Led sex Education)

The aim of RIPPLE is to improve the quality of teenage sexual relationships, reduce unsafe sex and reduce sexually transmitted infections and unwanted pregnancies. The delivery of RIPPLE is through peer educators from Year 13 working with students in Year 9.

The programme began in 1995 with the pilot phase being carried out over the first year. The trial continued until 2001 at point of publication and involves 27 coeducational comprehensive secondary schools in central southern England. The programme continues to be delivered in a number of schools.

Evaluation to date

In 1995–6 the pilot study took place in four schools to assess the feasibility of implementing the intervention.

During 1997–2001 there was a randomized trial of RIPPLE involving 27 schools. Main trial outcomes were assessed by questionnaire survey at baseline, 6, 12 and 24 months post-intervention. This was complemented by detailed process evaluation with pupils, teachers, peer educators and senior management.

Evaluation is ongoing at time of publication, with a follow-up of the trial to establish impact on terminations using NHS data.

Findings to date

The evaluation found high acceptability of the intervention to pupils, schools and peer educators, and positive impacts on knowledge and confidence of peer educators. To date the evaluation data available is limited but publications of results are forthcoming.

A PAUSE[3] (Added Power And Understanding in Sex Education)

The aims of A PAUSE are to enable young people to resist pressure either to have sex or unprotected sex until they judge the time to be right for them, while discouraging intolerance of those sexually active or of same-sex orientation, to enhance teacher's and health professionals' skills of delivery in collaborative learning styles and to

Box 11.2 (continued)

develop peers' interpersonal skills. It is hoped this can be achieved through a combined peer, teacher and health professional led sex education programme. Teachers and health professionals deliver sessions to Years 9 and 10 supported by sessions delivered by Year 12 peer educators. There is also an alternative Year 10 component delivered by Year 11 drama students as part of their GCSE curriculum.

In 1991 the research phase started in two intervention schools and 12 control schools. By 2003 the intervention was being delivered in over 140 schools spread around England and Wales (pre-intervention cohorts provide control groups for the evaluation). A nationally accredited qualification for peers was piloted in 2002–3 and a parallel peer delivered programme was re-piloted for use in schools exclusion units (2003–4).

Evaluation to date

This includes an Action Research Model with qualitative and quantitative evaluation continuously informing of programme developments.

There is process evaluation of Year 9 adult and peer-delivered sessions for data to schools on quality of delivery and perceptions of pupils. Peer assessment is also included.

Questionnaire assessment in Year 11 provides impact evaluation of the pupils' perceptions of the usefulness of their sex education, attitudes, beliefs and behaviours including age of first intercourse and use of contraception. In 2003 external evaluation was carried out of the whole programme by the National Foundation for Educational Research (NFER) on behalf of the Teenage Pregnancy Unit.

Findings to date

Findings from the NFER were not available at time of publication but previous evaluation found the programme was acceptable to all stakeholders, from pupils to governors, in a wide variety of school contexts varying from rural to inner city deprivation and from true comprehensives to Christian faith schools and those with high Muslim representation. It also found much higher ratings by pupils of their sex education and its usefulness in their lives. They demonstrated an increase in knowledge, sexually mature attitudes to relationships, realistic beliefs about age of and delay of actual first intercourse, and reduced rates of unprotected sex. There was no increase in intolerance to those either sexually active or of same-sex orientation.

and empathetic approach; positive attitudes and values towards sexual behaviour; a safe environment in which to deal openly with questions and concerns (Forrest *et al.*, 2002).

There are also practical considerations when delivering SRE in schools. For example, mixed classes are useful in terms of gender understanding but learning may be hindered by the pronounced differences in gender responses to the subject matter and materials. SHARE found that pupils, particularly boys, tended to censor discussion feedback when in mixed gender groups, and teachers found it more useful to use small mixed-gender groups of no more than four people (Wight *et al.*, 2000).

Young people indicate that they want SRE at school and it is important for this to continue. However, schools are increasingly seeing the benefits of delivering this in partnership with others, including parents, health promotion specialists, school health services, youth drop-in centres, churches and family planning agencies. Multi-agency approaches can have many benefits (Lowden and Pownie, 1994): for example, where 'outsiders' may be brought into schools to explore personal issues, with young people reassured in the knowledge that they will not see him/her again after the completion of the course. There are however issues relating to the sustainability of this approach.

Underpinning these considerations is the issue of training and support for teachers during initial teacher training and post qualification. The quality of initial teacher training with regard to health and SRE is currently varied, and it is possible in some institutions to graduate as a teacher without having taken an introductory course in this area. Although there are clearly other pressures on the training programme, this would be an ideal time to start to equip future teachers with skills and confidence in relation to SRE, and not doing so could be viewed as a wasted opportunity. In reality, post qualification training may be the most fertile area of development to improve the skills of teachers, although there are also pressures on time, resources and conflicting priorities for senior management. Evaluation from SHARE indicates high levels of confidence and increased competence following five days of intensive SRE training (Wight and Buston, in press).

Legal considerations for schools

The legal issues relevant to SRE are complex, particularly around confidentiality, which is a key concern for young people. Sex under 16 years is illegal and this creates difficulties for teachers who are bound by a professional code of conduct, which is also informed by ethical concerns, child protection guidelines and school policies. Health professionals are bound by their own code of conduct, whereby they are enabled to make professional judgments about the appropriateness of advice and maintaining confidentiality.

Inclusive SRE must address the issue of sexual diversity. However, many teachers have felt vulnerable raising the issue of homosexuality in the classroom given Section 28 of the Local Government Act 1986, which applied in England and Wales until 2003 and prohibited the promotion of homosexuality by teaching or published material. In Scotland this clause was repealed in 2000, and while a series of guidance and training was offered as part of the process, teachers are still unclear how to handle the issue in class. The clause has never applied in Northern Ireland.

Parents have the right to withdraw their children from any aspect of the curriculum, but are charged with the task of providing a suitable alternative. The same is true for SRE. However, the UN Convention on the Rights of the Child states that the views of the child should be taken into consideration if such a request is made. Given that aspects of relationships education permeate the curriculum it could be argued that withdrawal of a young person could interfere with his or her overall education opportunities.

Other differences exist between the countries: for example, in England and Wales, there is a statutory requirement for school governors to approve the SRE curriculum of the school (Green, 1994). In Scotland school boards do not have such powers, although there is now a requirement in Scotland that parents are consulted about the SRE programme of the school.

Moving into practice: developing a school policy

One practical way in which schools can move forward is to develop a policy for SRE, linking with key partners to encourage discussion and joint consideration of the issues laid out above. However, any policy should be developed with the following in mind:

- Education for sexuality and relationships is a lifelong process, and schools can contribute to this through nursery, primary and secondary education.
- Wider issues of health promotion outside the curriculum may convey messages as powerful as any learning and teaching in the classroom, as illustrated above.
- The way young people feel about school in general may be as important as any specific learning and teaching in the classroom. For example, there is some evidence that where there is conflict between young people and parents, if the former feel good about school then this is associated with a lower likelihood of being involved in high-risk behaviours, such as drinking excessively (Currie and Todd, 1993).
- SRE should be embedded in a wider health education or social education curriculum, as there are interconnections between various topics and themes; for example, the link between alcohol and drug use and high-risk behaviours, such as unprotected sex (Plant, 1990).
- SRE should explore emotions and practise skills, which are as important as acquiring knowledge and understanding about sex and relationships. For example, young people who have had unprotected sex leading to

pregnancy often state that they knew the risks but that their emotions overruled any reservations that they may have had.

- Learning and teaching relating to sexuality should build on young people's pre-existing knowledge and beliefs. To do this effectively, participatory learning methods should be employed to avoid assumptions about what pupils already know or about what issues they wish to know.
- School's influence is one of many and young people, as they mature, need the opportunity to explore the various beliefs and attitudes that may influence their behaviour. This could be particularly important in an area such as sex education, where informal sources of information are more important than, for example, in nutrition education, where the school and family are often the main sources of information (Young, 1992).
- Parental involvement can enhance effectiveness of health education programmes (Perry, 1988) and indeed is required by policy. The active cooperation of parents in the planning of SRE programmes can enhance the key partnership between home and school.
- School SRE needs to address gender issues apparent in the classroom, realizing that boys need education on issues such as sexual orientation and menstruation to counteract misconceptions and stereotyping. For many young males, school health education classes may be the only opportunity they have to learn about and discuss issues relating to sexuality and gender. The groups in the population most likely to report having unprotected sex are young, male and single (Johnson *et al.*, 1994).
- The effectiveness of aspects of school SRE will be increased by schools making links with other agencies, such as drop in centres or health centres where confidential advice is available.

Conclusion

This chapter shows how schools can play a key role in partnership with parents, school boards or governors, and specialist confidential services in improving the sexual health of young people.

However, a number of challenges exist, including fostering realistic expectations as to the role school SRE can play in changing behaviour and impacting on public health outcomes. It is difficult to expect schools to be the sole intervention to improve sexual health given the complex nature of sexuality and the range of factors from socioeconomic through to individual, which influence attitudes, beliefs and behaviour. Recent evaluations indicate that the success of SRE in schools may be best measured in educational outcomes (Wight *et al.*, 2002).

Partnership working to improve the quality and consistency of SRE in schools needs to continue and develop. There is a need to resolve the differences between the expectations of the education and health sectors in relation to sex and relationships education.

Finally, regardless of the deliverer in the classroom, SRE in schools should be teacher led: that is, the final responsibility of programme content and so on should rest within the school, and to do this teachers need to feel supported, confident and competent in their own skills if we are to ensure the quality of SRE continues to improve and meets the needs of young people in the future.

Notes

1 For more detail on SHARE see www.msoc-mrc.gla.ac.uk/Publications/ pub/share_MAIN.html
2 http://ioewebserver.ioe.ac.uk/ioe/cms/get.asp?cid=1509&1509_0=1513
3 www.ex.ac.uk/sshs/apause

References

Collins, C., Alagiri, P. and Summers, T. (2002) *Abstinence Only vs Comprehensive Sex Education: What are the Arguments? What is the Evidence?* AIDS Policy Research Center & Center for AIDS Prevention Studies, University of California, San Francisco.

Combes, G. (1989) The ideology of health education in schools. *British Journal of Sociology of Education* 10: 67–80.

CRD NHS (NHS Centre for Reviews and Dissemination) (1997) Preventing and reducing the adverse effects of unintended teenage pregnancies. *Effective Health Care* 3(1): 1–12.

Currie, C. and Todd, J. (1993) *Health Behaviours of Scottish Schoolchildren: Report 2 and Report 3.* University of Edinburgh: Research Unit in Health and Behavioural Change.

ten Dam, G.(2002) in I. Young (ed.), *Conference Report: Education and Health in Partnership,* World Health Organization Regional Office for Europe, 17–22.

Dixon, H. (2003) *SHARE (Sexual Health and Relationships Education) Training Manual.* Edinburgh: Health Education Board for Scotland.

Drew, S. (2000) *Children and the Human Rights Act 1998.* London: Save the Children.

Faculty of Public Health Medicine, Committee on Health Promotion Guidelines (1995) Sex education for young people: a background review. *Guidelines for Health Promotion* 42: 1–8. London: Faculty of Public Health Medicine.

Forrest, S., Strange, V. and Oakley, A. (2002) A comparison of students' evaluations of a peer-delivered sex education programme and teacher-led provision. *Sex Education* 2(3): 195–214.

Green, J. (1994) School governors and sex education: an analysis of policies in Leeds. *Health Education Journal,* 53: 40–51.

Johnson, A., Wadsworth, J., Wellings, K. and Field, J. (1994) *Sexual Attitudes and Lifestyles.* London: Blackwell Scientific.

Keogh, H. (1985) *The Inter-Relationship of Health and Education 1914–1946.* Ph.D. thesis, University of Manchester.

Kirby, D. (1997) *No Easy Answers: Research Findings on Programs to Reduce*

Teen Pregnancy. Washington, DC: National Campaign to Prevent Teen Pregnancy.

Kirby, D. (2001) *Emerging Answers: Research Findings on Programmes to Reduce Unwanted Teenage Pregnancy.* Washington, DC: National Campaign to Prevent Teen Pregnancy.

Lewis, D. (1993) Oh for those halcyon days! A review of the development of school health education over 50 years. *Health Education Journal,* **52**:161–71.

Lowden, K. and Pownie, J. (1994) *Drugs, Alcohol and Sex Education. A Report of Two Innovative School Based Programmes.* Scottish Council for Research in Education.

Meyrick, J. and Swann, C. (1998) *An Overview of the Effectiveness of Interventions and Programmes Aimed at Reducing Unintended Conceptions in Young People.* London: Health Education Authority.

National Board of Education (1939) *Suggestions on Health Education.* London: HMSO.

Perry, C. (1988) Parent involvement with children's health promotion: the Minnesota Home Team. *American Journal of Public Health* **78**:11156–60

Plant, M. (1990) Alcohol, sex and AIDS. *Journal of Alcohol and Alcoholism* **25**: 293–301.

Power, P. (1995) Menstrual complexities. *Health Education* **2**: 17–21.

Rogers, E. M. (1962) *The Diffusion of Innovations.* New York: Free Press.

Scottish Consultative Council on the Curriculum (1999) *Curriculum Design for the Secondary Stages: Guidelines for Schools.* Scottish CCC, 7–9.

UNAIDS (1997) *Impact of HIV and Sexual Health Education on the Sexual Behaviour of Young People.* Joint United Nations Programme on HIV/AIDS.

Wellings, K., Wadsworth, J., Johnson, A. M., Field, J., Whitaker, L. and Field, B. (1995) Provision of sex education and early sexual experience: the relationship examined. *British Medical Journal* **311**: 417–20.

Wight, D. and Abraham, C. (2000) From psycho-social theory to sustainable classroom practice: developing a research-based teacher-delivered sex education programme. *Health Education Research: Theory and Practice* **15**: 25–38.

Wight, D. and Buston, K. (in press) Meeting the needs but not changing the goals: evaluation of in-service teacher training for sex education. *Oxford Review of Education.*

Wight, D., Raab, G., Henderson, M., Abraham, C., Buston, K., Hart, G. and Scott, S. (2002) Limits of teacher delivered sex education: interim behavioural outcomes from a randomised trial, *British Medical Journal* **324**, 15 June: 1430–5.

Young, I. (1992) *A Study of the Effects of a School Health Promotion Initiative on the Knowledge, Attitudes and Behaviour of the Pupils.* M.Ph. thesis, University of Glasgow.

Young, I. (1993) Healthy eating policies in schools: an evaluation of pupils' knowledge, attitudes and behaviour. *Health Education Journal,* **52**: 3–9.

Young, I. and Williams, T. (1989) *The Healthy School.* Scottish Health Education Group/World Health Organization Regional Office for Europe.

12 Communication and Sex Education in Families

AUDREY SIMPSON

> **Key issues**
>
> - Parents in the UK are less likely than parents in most other European countries to discuss sex and relationships with their children.
> - The family environment plays a significant part in determining sexual health outcomes.
> - Health educators must provide parents with information and communication skills to enable them to talk more openly about sexual issues with their children.

Overview

This chapter examines the influence of parents and the role they can play in educating their children about sexuality, identifying a range of barriers that can limit parental action and their impact as sex educators. While the chapter will focus mostly on communication and ways to improve this, it will also touch on the importance of broader family experiences on developing sexuality. Speakeasy, a project based in Northern Ireland, is used to highlight ways in which parents can be supported to develop the skills necessary to discuss sexual matters with their children. The issues relating to children not in traditional family or parental situations are discussed in a separate chapter.

Introduction

As far back as the early nineteenth century, providing information about sex and relationships was regarded as the domain of the home and, to a lesser extent, the church. A strong moral line on sex only within marriage was promoted, and for women in particular sex was often portrayed as something necessary in terms of wifely duty and procreation rather than as something to actively participate in and enjoy. The specifics of sex and issues of sexual pleasure and negotiation were rarely discussed: brides-to-be told simply to 'lie back and think of England!' (Dallas, 1972; Rogers, 1974).

During the twentieth century the perceived importance and relevance of effective sex education grew, partly in acknowledgement of the fact that parents were not adequately equipping their children with the necessary information about sex and sexuality. Schools were identified to take some responsibility for sex education (National Board of Education, 1943) supplementing the crucial role of parents (Newsom Report, 1963; Church of England, 1964), and by the 1980s school-based sex education was well established and built into the school curriculum in some areas of the UK (although not without professional and political concerns over content, quality and consistency).

Despite these changes and the broader cultural shift since the 1960s towards more liberal attitudes to sexuality and sexual lifestyles, some parents still struggle to communicate with their children about sexual matters. Recent sexual health policy has reflected both the importance of parents as sex educators and the discomfort and lack of confidence (or even basic knowledge) that many parents feel. Both the SEU teenage pregnancy report (SEU, 1999) and the Northern Irish action plan on teenage pregnancy (DHSSPS, 2002) emphasize the importance of parents in helping children and young people to cope with their developing sexuality and to develop relationships that are based on respect for themselves and others. At the same time, work directly supporting and advising parents is increasing across the UK, recognizing the wide range of needs of individual parents and children and working with sensitivity to cultural and religious differences.

Why parents are important

Before moving into this discussion, it is important to recognize that parents are a diverse group. They will come from different cultures, background and religious groups. Parenting also takes many forms. For example, they may be single, coupled, married, divorced, heterosexual, bisexual, lesbian, and may be natural, adoptive or foster. However the information in this chapter applies to anyone assuming a parental role, whatever that may look like specifically.

Primary influencers

Parents are the primary influences on their children and have a profound impact on their developing beliefs, attitudes and behaviours. Theories of socialization, social learning and identity formation (for example, Bandura, 1977) describe how children in particular internalize parental attitudes and often act in response to parental behaviour (whether consistent or deliberately at odds with this behaviour). In relation to sexuality and relationships, Porter (1991) argues that these are first nurtured in the home. Children learn and are consciously and unconsciously shaped both by what parents tell them directly and by observing how parents talk and act in their own relationships with partners and others. In this way, anyone in a parenting relationship is educating their child about sexuality, even if they are not directly teaching the 'facts of life'.

Learning about gender and gender roles and expectations is a vital element of developing sexuality (McDonald and Parke, 1986; Robinson and Morris, 1986). Even before a child enters school she/he will already have a strong sense of female or male identity. Jackson (1982), in her examination of children's experiences on the way to sexual maturity, pointed out:

> The aspect of early development which has the greatest impact on our sexuality is not specifically sexual. It is through learning about gender – discovering the significance according to the differences between the sexes, and developing a sense of themselves as feminine or masculine – that children begin to develop a basis for later sexual learning. Girls and boys learn to be sexual in different ways and it is in childhood, when they begin to learn to think and act in accordance with our ideals of femininity and masculinity, that the foundations of these different styles of sexuality are built.
>
> (Jackson, 1982: 79)

Family environment

The broad socioeconomic context of the family, in particular the social class and education levels of parents, is important in shaping the values and expectations of children. It also influences sexual health outcomes; for example, young women from poorer backgrounds are more likely to become pregnant in their teenage years and to continue with the pregnancy (see Chapter 2). The influence of class and education is in part via expectations and social norms, which make early sexual activity and parenthood more acceptable and less likely to impact on long-term aspirations in some communities that in others.

In addition, as other chapters in this book discuss, religious (moral) and ethnic factors influence the norms and expectations communicated and fostered within families, and in turn impact on sexual attitudes and behaviour (Thornton and Camburn, 1987).

General family structure and history are also linked to sexual health outcomes. For example, Newcomer and Udry (1985) identified a clear relationship between a mother's sexual experience as a teenager and the sexual experience of her daughter; they also showed that girls from single-parent families are more likely to become sexually active at an earlier age than those from a two-parent family. Further, the daughter of a teenage mother is one and half times more likely to become one herself than the daughter of an older mother (SEU, 1999).

Family dynamics, for example time spent together in family activities, parental support, behaviour control/parental monitoring and family conflict also shape attitudes and behaviour. Time spent in family activities (Sweeting *et al.*, 1998) and parental support or connectedness with children (Chewning and Koningsfeld, 1998; Feldman and Brown, 1993; Jaccard *et al.*, 1996; Resnick *et al.*, 1997) are associated with later age at first intercourse and reduced sexual activity. In addition, parental acceptance increases self-esteem, which is linked to reduced likelihood of teenage pregnancy (Emler, 2001).

Findings from SHARE (Wight *et al.*, in press) showed that for young men, greater parental monitoring and lower spending money (at first data collection point) were associated with less sexual experience and lower number of sexual partners (spending money only) two years later. For young women, higher parental monitoring was associated with later sexual experience, lower numbers of sexual partners and greater condom and contraceptive use. A similar pattern emerged for low spending money (with the exception of contraception and condom use).

Patterns of communication in families are another important influence on sexual health attitudes and behaviour relating to sexual health. Good communication facilitates discussion about sex and is often the focus of health promotion activity, not least because of the potential for influence and change. The remainder of this chapter will focus on this issue.

Talking about sex
Why talking matters

Discussions about sex have a direct impact on sexual health decisions. Some studies have indicated that family discussion about sexual matters is related to higher levels of knowledge about sexuality and lower incidence of sexual risk-taking behaviour (Fisher, 1989; Pick and Palos, 1995). Those who had discussed sex were more likely to delay first intercourse (Dilorio *et al.*, 1999; Mitchell and Wellings, 1998; Casper, 1990; Taris *et al.*, 1998), and when sex did occur, to use contraception (Wellings *et al.*, 2001; Schubotz *et al.*, 2002). Research from Northern Ireland showed that only 17.3 per cent of young men who did not use contraception at first sex found it easy to talk to their mothers about sexual matters, compared with over 30 per cent of those who did use some form of contraception (Schubotz *et al.*, 2002). Those young people who did not use any contraception found it hardest to talk to their fathers about sex. These findings are similar to Scottish data (Todd *et al.*, 1999) indicating that boys who have discussed contraception with parents feel more comfortable about carrying condoms.

What parents currently discuss

Parents in the UK are less likely than those in some other countries to talk to their children about sex (SEU, 1999). Although many parents recognize that they have a responsibility, this does not always result in action. Ingham (2002) found significant differences between recognition of responsibility and what happens in practice. For example, 93 per cent of parents said they should discuss contraception but only 29 per cent had done so; 92 percent said that they should discuss abortion compared with 40 per cent who had actually done so (Table 12.1).

The Health Promotion Agency for Northern Ireland (1996) found that only 25 per cent of parents had discussed contraception with their children and only 19 per cent had discussed abortion. The biggest criticism from young people in the 2002 Northern Ireland survey was parents' reluctance to discuss feelings and emotions, including potentially contentious subjects such as sexual orientation or how to make sex more satisfying (Schubotz *et al.*, 2002). Explanations were frequently lacking – warnings to 'be careful' and 'just watch yourself' were common but what they had to 'be careful about' was not elaborated upon. Parents confirmed that they rarely discussed sex-related topics with their children:

> My girls never came home and talked to me. If I knew say they had a film in school they came home and I said, 'Well what happened?' 'Oh this and that and the other.' I said, 'Well have you any questions?' 'No!' My girls have never come with questions except when they were younger, you know, wee tiny silly questions. After that they never came and asked questions. To be honest I don't know what I would have done if they had so I suppose it was a bit of a relief.

Young people seem fully aware of the taboo nature of talking about sex with their parents, commenting on the embarrassment, lack of knowledge and difference in attitudes as a result of the age difference:

Table 12.1 Parental views of responsibility and parental action in relation to discussion with their children (%)

Topic	Responsibility	Action
Saying 'no'	97	47
The role of emotions	95	48
Contraception	95	58
Abuse and rape	93	50
Discussing contraception with partner	93	29
Abortion	92	40
HIV/AIDS	91	60
Values	91	49
Homosexuality	90	52

Source: Ingham, 2002

See probably half the time our parents don't know about contraception or what, they might still have some sex life but not an awful lot.

(Speakeasy project)

Influences on discussion

The main influences on communication about sexuality between parents and children that have been explored in the literature are parenting style, parental attitudes to sex, and sexuality and gendered interaction between parent and child.

Parenting style

Three parenting styles have been identified: authoritative, authoritarian and permissive (Shucksmith and Hendry, 1998; Foxcroft and Lowe, 1995). Typically those who adopt a more authoritative style are likely to discuss issues, including sexual health matters (Aggleton *et al.*, 1998; Ingham, 2002), rather than to dictate behaviour as in the authoritarian style. If discussion of sexual matters is done in a skilled and comfortable manner it may promote discussion about sex with a partner (Whitaker *et al.*, 1999). The permissive style provides neither control nor support; along with the authoritarian style it is linked to problem behaviour (Foxcroft and Lowe, 1995).

Parental attitudes to sex

Parental attitudes specifically towards adolescent sexual behaviour are important for how and what they communicate to their children. While some parents are happy to discuss sex within the family, others are less willing, often because of their own experiences. Table 12.2 illustrates some of the difficulties parents face.

The following account from the real experiences of one parent grappling with sex education graphically illustrates the feelings of embarrassment and avoidance tactics employed:

'Mummy what is a lesbian?' (10 year old daughter)
'Where did you hear that word?' (mother, uncomfortable, embarrassed)
'Well, Zoe in Emmerdale is a lesbian.' (daughter)
'Oh yes. Well now, a lesbian is a female vet.' (mother, very relieved)

Parental values and how these are expressed in families are also key. For example, FPA Northern Ireland's experience of working with women faced with an unplanned pregnancy revealed that those who choose not to tell their parents about their pregnancy are those whose parents have been very vocal in their condemnation of sex outside marriage.

Table 12.2 Barriers to communication identified by parents

Quotes from parents	Barrier identified
It would encourage them to have sex.	Poor knowledge.
It's too personal.	Taboo subject.
I don't know where to start.	No role model.
I don't know what words to use.	Lack of confidence and knowledge.
My child doesn't have feelings like that.	Denial.
My mother would kill me.	Family background.
I wasn't told anything and I got by.	Cultural attitudes.
I would die.	Embarrassment.

Source: Speakeasy project

Gendered interaction

There are clear gender differences in parent/child communication. Mothers tend to be the main educators in the household regardless of whether the children are sons or daughters (Walker, 2001; Feldman and Rosenthal, 2000; Nolin and Petersen, 1992). Fathers are less likely to be involved in sex education. In general, children view it as more important for mothers than fathers to communicate about sexual matters (Rosenthal and Feldman, 1999).

The 2002 Northern Ireland survey showed that young women were much more likely than young men to receive information from their mothers. They were also almost three times as likely as young men to say that this information was the most helpful to them. Young men also learnt more from their mothers, but were more than twice as likely as young women to receive some sex education from their fathers.

This is consistent with a more general finding that mothers are likely to take on the responsibility of interpersonal relations in the family, and are likely to deal with personal issues in a less judgemental manner than fathers (Noller and Callan, 1991). Mothers appear to be more comfortable talking to daughters about physical development and relationships, relating to this by thinking about their own sexual development (Walker, 2001).

Supporting parents

It is clear that many parents do not do all that they can in relation to the formal as opposed to informal transmission of sexual knowledge, even though young people would like them to (MacDowall *et al.*, 2002). It is important to explore the reasons behind this in order to be able to encourage and enable parents to take a more active role in this arena.

Approaches for supporting parents vary from policy level initiatives to community-led projects. For example, guidance for the development of school-based sex education policy stipulates consultation with parents as a key element. In Scotland Healthy Respect, a government-funded long-term initiative to improve the sexual health of young people, works with parents to develop age-specific materials. Other examples of community based initiatives can be found across the UK, but of particular interest is Speakeasy, a project first established in Northern Ireland by the FPA and subsequently adopted in other parts of the UK (see Box 12.1).

Conclusion

Parents, directly and indirectly, play an important role in shaping and influencing the behaviour and attitudes of young people with regard to sex, sexuality and gender. However many parents, no matter how caring and supportive, are still reluctant to assume responsibility for the direct sex education of their children. This chapter argues that many parents are committed to helping their children cope with their developing sexuality but simply lack the relevant confidence, information and skills to do this effectively. Practical community-based programmes designed with sensitivity to local needs offer a means of providing the required support to parents. But such work should not be confined to a box marked 'sex education'. It is just as much about family support (improved relationships within families), health issues (parents are more informed about their own health and are more likely to access services), personal development (skills and confidence building of the parents) and community development (addresses social inclusion). This ties in with the more holistic concept of health promotion that many experienced practitioners in this field endorse as opposed to a narrow focus on 'nuts and bolts' and the biological realities of sex.

Box 12.1 Speakeasy project

Speakeasy is a community development project, which is based on the ethos of participant ownership and influence. It is based on the rights of children and young people to have information and support regarding their sexuality. It involves six to eight weekly workshops, which are person centred, needs led, and confidential. As a course, it is accredited up to Level Two through the Northern Ireland Open College Network. The project aims to encourage parents to provide positive sex education in the home by giving them the necessary support and information to take on the role of sex educator. Parents are offered the opportunity to increase their levels of information and confidence in three areas:

Box 12.1 continued

- skills relating to talking to children about sex
- knowledge of sexual health
- personal and cultural attitudes and values towards sex education.

External evaluation of Speakeasy (FPA NI, 1998) found that as a result of the course parents were convinced of the importance of children and young people getting clear information about sex, sexuality and relationships. They recognized the crucial role of parents in sexual socialization, and accepted that avoidance had been giving powerful messages to their children by presenting sex and sexuality as taboo subjects. Virtually without exception parents felt that their own parents had not informed them adequately about sexual matters and that they were in danger of repeating the same patterns. In particular the evaluation highlighted:

- improved relationships between parent and child
- improved relationship with partner
- enhanced individual capacity building around confidence and parenting skills
- increased level of personal knowledge
- community capacity building as health and community workers later reported community impetus.

As with other projects of this type, it was difficult to attract men to participate in Speakeasy. However, male recruitment improved in the second Speakeasy project, probably linked to a growing interest in Northern Ireland in men's health issues and the concept of masculinity. The introduction of men brought challenges, as there was a reluctance to acknowledge their needs to explore feelings towards sex before talking about such issues with their children, but it turned out to be a positive experience.

In 1999 funding was secured to establish a second Speakeasy in Derry, running as a cross-border initiative with County Donegal in the Republic of Ireland. Despite cultural and religious differences, Speakeasy provided participants with the opportunity to share universal concerns and problems as parents. In 2001 the project was implemented by FPA UK in several areas in England.

One parent who participated in Speakeasy poignantly illustrates the importance of parents in the sex education of children. When preparing a collage of useful contact numbers for teenagers she cut out an advertisement from a teen magazine. The advert was for a young person's help line. The mother drew a bold line through the advert and replaced it with the following words:

I am my child's help line!

References

Aggleton, P., Oliver, C. and Rivers, K. (1998) *The Implications of Research into Young People, Sex, Sexuality and Relationships*. London: Health Education Authority.

Bandura, A. (1977) Self-efficacy: toward a unifying theory of behavioural change. *Psychological Review* **84**: 191–215.

Casper, L. M. (1990) Does family interaction prevent adolescent pregnancy? *Family Planning Perspectives* **22**(3): 109–14.

Chewning, B. and Koningsfeld, R. V. (1998) Predicting adolescent's initiation of intercourse and contraceptive use. *Journal of Applied Social Psychology* **28**(14): 1245–85.

Church of England Board of Education (1964) *Sex Education in Schools*. London: Church Information Office.

Dallas, D. (1972) *Sex Education in School and Society*. National Foundation for Education Research.

DHSSPS (2002) *Teenage Pregnancy and Parenthood. Strategy and Action Plan 2002–2007*. Belfast.

DiIorio, C., Kelley, M. and Hockenberry-Eaton, M. (1999) Communication about sexual issues: mothers, fathers and friends. *Journal of Adolescent Health* **24**(3): 181–9.

Emler, N. (2001) *Self-Esteem: The Costs and Causes of Low Self-Worth*. York: Joseph Rowntree Foundation.

Feldman, S. and Brown, N. (1993) Family influences on adolescent male sexuality: the mediation role of self-restraint. *Social Development* **2**: 15–35.

Feldman, S. and Rosenthal, D. (2000) The effects of communication characteristics on family members' perceptions of parents as sex educators. *Journal of Research on Adolescence* **10**(2): 119–50.

Fisher, T. D. (1989) An extension of the findings of Moore, Peterson and Furstenberg (1986) regarding family sexual communication and adolescent sexual behaviour. *Journal of Marriage and the Family* **51**(3): 637–9.

Foxcroft, D. and Lowe, G. (1995) Adolescent drinking, smoking and other substance use involvement: links with perceived family life. *Journal of Adolescence* **18**: 159–77.

FPA (1998) *Evaluation of Speakeasy Project* (unpublished), Belfast: FPA.

Health Promotion Agency for Northern Ireland (1996) *Sex Education in Northern Ireland: Views from Parents and Schools*. Belfast: HPA.

Ingham, R. (2002) *The Role of Parents in Sex Education. Young People and Sexual Health: Report of a Deliberative Seminar*. HEBS, Edinburgh.

Jaccard, J., Dittus, P. J. and Gordon, V. V. (1996) Maternal correlates of adolescent sexual and contraceptive behavior. *Family Planning Perspectives* **28**: 159–65.

Jackson, S. (1982) *Childhood and Sexuality*. Oxford: Blackwell.

MacDowall, W., Gerrassu, M., Nanchahal, K. and Wellings, K. (2002) *Analysis of Natsal 2000 Data for Scotland*. Edinburgh: Health Education Board for Scotland.

McDonald, K. and Parke, R. D. (1986) Parent–child physical play. *Sex Roles* **15**: 367–78.

Milburn, K. (1996) *Peer Education: Young People and Sexual Health, a Critical Review*. Working Paper Number 2, Edinburgh: Health Education Board for Scotland.

Mitchell, K. and Wellings, K. (1998) First sexual intercourse: anticipation and communication: interviews with young people in England. *Journal of Adolescence* **21**(6): 717–26.

National Board of Education (1943) Sex education in schools and youth organisations, in M. Hill and L. Jones (1970) *Sex Education – The Erroneous Zone*. National Secular Society.

Newsom Report (1953) *Half Our Future*. London: HMSO.

Newcomer, S. F. and Udry, R. (1985) Parent child communication and adolescent sexual behaviour. *Family Planning Perspectives* **17**(4).

Nolin, M. J. and Petersen, K. K. (1992) Gender differences in parent–child communication about sexuality, *Journal of Adolescent Research*, 7.

Noller, P. and Callan, V. (1991) *The Adolescent in the Family*. London: Routledge.

Pick, S. and Palos, P. (1995) Impact of the family on the sex lives of adolescents. *Adolescence* **30**(119): 667–75.

Porter, M. (1991) *Sex Education Programmes for Parents*. World Health Organization.

Resnick, M. D., Bearman, P., Blum, R. W., Bauman, K. E., Harris, K. M., Jones, J., Tabor, J., Beuhring, T., Sieving, R. E., Shew, M., Ireland, M., Bearinger, L. H. and Udry, J. R. (1997) Protecting adolescents from harm: findings from the National Longitudinal Study on Adolescent Health. *Journal of American Medical Association* **278**(10): 823–32.

Robinson, C. C. and Morris, J. J. (1986) The gender-stereotyped nature of Christmas toys. *Sex Roles* 15: 21–32.

Rogers, R. (1974) *Sex Education: Rationale and Reaction*. Cambridge: Cambridge University Press.

Rosenthal, D. and Feldman, S. (1999) The importance of importance: parent–adolescent communication about sexuality. *Journal of Adolescence* 22: 835–52.

Schubotz, D., Simpson, A. and Rolston, B. (2002) *Towards Better Sexual Health: A Survey of Sexual Attitudes and Lifestyles of Young People in Northern Ireland*. London: FPA.

Shucksmith, J. and Hendry, L. B. (1998) *Health Issues and Adolescents: Growing Up, Speaking Out*. London: Routledge.

Social Exclusion Unit (SEU) (1999) *Teenage Pregnancy*. London: The Stationery Office.

Sweeting, H., West, P. and Richards, M. (1998) Teenage family life, lifestyles and life chances: associations with family structure, conflict with parents and joint family activity. *International Journal of Law, Policy and the Family* 12: 15–46.

Taris, T. W., Semin, G. R. and Bok, I. A. (1998) The effect of quality of family interaction and intergenerational transmission of values on sexual permissiveness. *Journal of Psychology* **159**(2): 237–50.

Thornton, A. and Camburn, D. (1987) The influence of the family on premarital sexual behaviour and attitudes. *Demography* 24: 323–40.

Todd, J., Currie, C. and Smith, R. (1999) *Health Behaviours of Scottish Schoolchildren, Technical Report 2: Sexual Health in the 1990s*. University of Edinburgh: Research Unit in Health and Behavioural Change.

Walker, J. L. (2001) A qualitative study of parents' experiences of providing sex education for their children: The implications for health education. *Health*

Education Journal **60**(2): 132–46.

Wellings, K., Nanchahal, K., Macdowall, W., McManus, S., Erens, B., Mercer, C. H., Johnson, A. M., Copas, A. J., Korovessis, C., Fenton, K. A. and Field, J. (2001) Sexual behaviour in Britain: early heterosexual experience. *The Lancet* 358: 1843–50.

Whitaker, D. J., Miller, K. S., May, D. C. and Levin, M. L. (1999) Teenage partners' communication about sexual risk and condom use: the importance of parent–teenage discussions. *Family Planning Perspectives* **31**(3): 117–21.

Wight, D., Williamson, L. and Henderson, M. (in press) *Parental Influences on Young People's Sexual Behaviour.*

13 'They Treated Us Like One of Them Really': Peer Education as an Approach to Sexual Health Promotion with Young People

SIMON FORREST

> **Key issues**
>
> - Peer education approaches to sex and relationships education (SRE) have received significant endorsement through UK government policy, and have been widely adopted despite limited evidence of their effectiveness.
> - In part the appeal of this approach is the participation nature of peer education to professionals in health, education and welfare services, although the extent to which power is really devolved or equitably shared with young people is questionable.
> - There is evidence to suggest that peer-led sex education is accessible and satisfactory to young people, and that peer educators benefit those involved in terms of personal development.

Overview

This chapter explores the potential strengths and weaknesses of peer education with young people. While there is particular reference to sexual health the majority of the chapter draws on evidence from a range of health topics, given the limited robust evidence base for peer education in sexual health specifically.

It first considers the policy context for sexual health peer education before examining the broader history and definitions of peer education, drawing on other health-related topics before discussing the effectiveness, usefulness and potential challenges of the approach. This chapter does not provide a comprehensive account of the organization and implementation of peer education projects.

Introduction

Peer education involving young people blossomed in the UK during the mid-1980s when it was perceived as one way of mobilizing communities to design and implement HIV/AIDS prevention schemes which were responsive and receptive to social and local norms and factors. The majority of projects seem to have been developed and to have operated at a local level, often initiated and supported by health promotion services. Youth and community services, where experience of youth involvement in informal and peer approaches to education and personal development was widespread and longstanding, contributed. Despite no systematic support for peer education it is believed that during this period more projects existed in the UK than the rest of Europe combined (Svenson, 1998).

In addition, while schools had been identified to deliver sex education, the shortage of trained, competent and confident staff suggested that peer education could access young people in relevant forms and through credible intermediaries. It also offered the possibility of maximizing returns in that training a few peer educators could provide the human resource to reach a wide group of young people. Peer education as a means of sex education and sexual health promotion with young people had, and still has, a political 'edge' which appeals to some professionals in health and education, and organizations that were keen to react to the problems of 'top-down' approaches.

More recently government policy initiatives have highlighted the potential for using peer education approaches to improve sex education in schools. For example, the teenage pregnancy strategy (Social Exclusion Unit, 1999) recommended peer education in schools and other settings with a particular potential to reach and involve young people in groups that are at risk. This focus has been reiterated in the guidance on SRE handed down to all maintained schools in England and Wales (DfEE, 2000). Explicit reference is made to the use of teenage parents and British Asian young people as peer educators, able respectively, to bring to life the realities of teenage parenthood and pitch sex education in ways that are appropriate to specific cultural and religious sensitivities. This has been followed by more detailed guidance on the process of setting up peer education projects using others' experience (Crosier *et al.*, 2002).

However peer education remains as susceptible as other approaches to societal difficulties with discussing sex and sexuality openly. 'Moralism' and continuing prejudice and inequality around gender and sexuality not only provide a poor basis on which to deal with sexual health issues but may also place limits on what peer educators are allowed or feel that they can do, particularly in formal settings like schools. In addition, the evidence base for peer education, while growing, is limited with regard to sexual health. Therefore this chapter will focus on the approach of peer education, drawing on a range of health related research and highlighting the issues for sexual health specifically where appropriate.

History of peer education

Early forms of peer education, like the monitorial system in Victorian schools, involved older school pupils teaching younger pupils to read and write, and was instituted to enable teachers to cope with large groups of children. Far from exploiting similarities between peer educators and their peers, the system positioned monitors as teachers in their own right with the power to dispense punishment and reward.

Peer education experienced a renaissance during the 1960s when it was widely termed peer tutoring. 'Tutoring' described the interaction between older students who provided learning support to their younger peers. Some educational psychologists (for example, Vygotsky, 1962) highlighted the benefits of equitable peer interaction in terms of internalization of learning. They posited that peer tutoring would help assimilation of new information and skills because the interaction would tap into normal cognitive processes which were stimulated by sharing thoughts, discussing things and learning to compromise with each other. Evaluation found that peer interaction also lacked the intimidating overtones children felt existed in their interactions within adult teachers, and that peer tutoring could contribute to creative thinking, help boost the motivation and self-esteem of underachieving pupils, and be a constructive social experience.

Peer counselling approaches were derived from this work. These focus on helping young people deal with their personal problems by putting them in contact with peers who have dealt with similar experiences. Both peer tutoring and counselling programmes are still used to promote literacy and numeracy and to work with young people in special circumstances, for example, those who have serious illnesses or are homeless.

Defining peer education

Definitions and emphasis of approach reflect the professional and academic perspectives of their originators and the social, political and cultural context in which they worked. Some definitions of peer education emphasize its role as a means of mobilizing young people; others place emphasis on the relationship between peer educators and their peers. Box 13.1 shows some commonly used definitions.

If we try to aggregate the essence of these definitions we can conclude that peer education is about effecting change in attitudes, values, knowledge, awareness and/or behaviour within a relatively homogenous group of people through the benign influence of members of that group. The similarities between the peer educators and peer educated mean that this transfer takes places efficiently, using existing social connections and networks in relevant and meaningful ways, and pitched at a level which is developmentally appropriate to the group.

The search for definitions has contributed to the formation of a complex taxonomy of peer-led approaches. Figure 13.1 synthesizes elements of three

---

Box 13.1 Definitions of peer education

Young people teaching other young people.

Clements and Buczkiewicz (1993)

Interaction between individuals with shared characteristics such as behaviour, experience, status or social and cultural backgrounds.

Charleston et al. (1998)

The sharing or teaching of health information, values and behaviours by members of similar age or status groups.

Sciacca (1987)

An approach whereby a minority of peer representatives from a group or population actively attempt to inform and influence the majority.

Svenson (1998)

An approach which empowers young people to work with other young people, and which draws on the positive strength of the peer group. By means of appropriate training and support the young people become active players in the educational process rather than the passive recipients of a set message.

Jaquet et al. (1996)

---

important and commonly used taxonomies, and draws on the views of three authors (Backes *et al.*, 2001; Hartley-Brewer, 2002; Svenson, 1998).

This complex model in part reflects the dynamic nature of work and difficulties with allocating projects to single categories. Nonetheless, it is important to begin to classify distinctions and this chapter will focus on those activities which are termed 'peer education'.

Theoretical basis of peer education

The lack of a clear theoretical basis for peer education has been one major criticism of the approach (Milburn, 1996). The proximity of peers in terms of age and/or their social status is at the root of all attempts to develop this basis and to generate hypotheses about how it functions. These characteristics of age and status similarity are reflected in a variety of psychosocial theories about health-related behaviour, learning and social influence (for example, Abraham and Sheeran, 1994; Wight *et al.*, 1998), which are usually employed to describe and explain how peer education approaches can effect change in young people's health-related knowledge, attitudes, skills and behaviour.

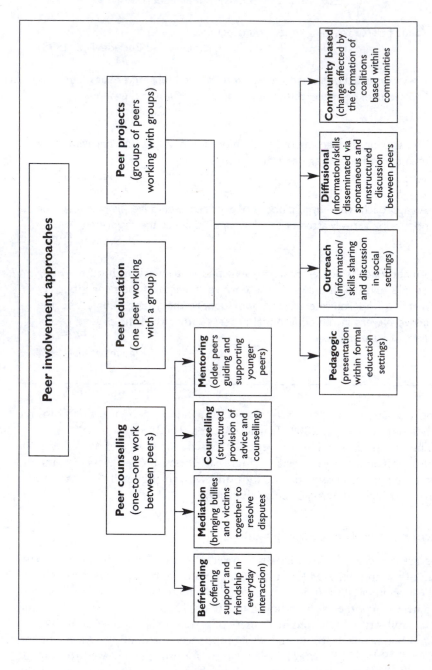

Figure 13.1 Taxonomies of approaches to peer involvement

Most theoretical explanations of peer education comprise three strands: theories or models which account for changes in health-related behaviour (Health Belief Model; Theory of Reasoned Action, and so on); theories on the role of social learning in cognitive, social and behavioural development; and theories on the transmission of new ideas, cultures or norms through social groups. Further discussion of how these models apply to peer education can be found elsewhere.

Of course, even by compounding theories it is not possible to foresee what will determine sexual behaviour, given the complexity of the interaction and dependence on situational factors. Therefore the effect of peer-led activity will be unpredictable, but may get closer to enabling young people to deal with the complexity, as they are highly influenced by perceptions of social norms and susceptible to peer influence (Campenhoudt *et al.*, 1997).

Peer education in health promotion

Peer education has potential for health promotion as it can tap into existing social networks and involve members of the target group who are accepted and accessible to their peers. It can also provide opportunities for cognitive, emotional and social development which comes from encouraging young people to take charge of their health and supporting them in protecting and improving the health of their peers (Weare, 2000). This involvement may help in the development of emotional literacy and high self-esteem, which are thought to underpin the achievement and maintenance of good health.

Peer education has potential particularly for sexual health because it meets the criteria for effective sex education particularly well, as it can fulfil requirements for sex education to begin early, before behaviour is established and resistant to change.

Effectiveness of peer education in health promotion

There is controversy about how to determine the effectiveness and impact of peer education activity, linked to methodology, design, quality and consistency of evaluation. However these issues are overtaken by the fact that a large number of peer education projects are never evaluated. Indeed the only randomized controlled trial (RCT) of peer-led sex education in the UK is the RIPPLE trial, so the body of research to which we can refer that meets the minimum requirements to be useful in assessing effectiveness is very small.

An important review of peer education was published in 1999 (Harden *et al.*). It aimed to critically examine the claim that the approach is a more effective and appropriate way of promoting young people's health than other traditional approaches. The review identified reports and papers relating to 271 separate interventions, most of which took place in the USA (68 per cent) and a few in the UK (15 per cent).

Twelve of the reports met the review criteria and contributed to the assessment of the effectiveness; eight related to in-school programmes. Two of the interventions included had a sexual health focus while the remainder targeted smoking prevention, testicular examination and aggressive male behaviour.

Impact on knowledge, attitudes and behaviour

Seven studies showed that peer education changed young people's behaviour, and all the rest bar one showed an increase in knowledge, positive shifts in attitudes and behavioural intentions or self efficacy. The two studies which focused on HIV or STI prevention both took place in college settings and showed positive changes in young people's knowledge and attitudes, self efficacy and their intention to practise safer sex.

Community versus school setting

In community settings both educational and community mobilization approaches were found to be effective at influencing the sexual behaviour of young people in their late teens. One programme increased condom use among African-American young women and another reduced unprotected anal intercourse among young gay men. Formal programmes in school settings tended to focus on social influence, and those outside school involved working with the wider social and cultural determinants of health-related behaviour.

Peer versus teacher-led activity

Five of the studies compared a peer education approach to teachers delivering the same programme. In two of these peer education was more effective, in two as effective, and in one neither the teachers nor peer educators were effective. Mellanby *et al.* (2000) have looked specifically at research that compares peer-led and adult-led health education in schools and found 13 studies, predominantly relating to programmes implemented in schools in North America. These programmes were similarly diverse to those identified by Harden and her colleagues in terms of the range of topics addressed.

Eleven of the studies looked at how the programme impacted on young people's behaviour. Seven showed peer educators to be more effective than teachers in the long term and the remaining four found no difference between peer educators and teachers. All 11 studies also compared the effects of programmes provided by peer educators and teachers to other groups of young people. In this comparison peer education was more effective in nine studies (although only with girls in one of them) and teachers in four.

Although these reviews do suggest that peer education can be effective, both research teams noted that it was difficult to identify the characteristics that made the approach effective because the pool of studies was small, the range of topics addressed diverse, the young people involved differed greatly in age and backgrounds, and because reports did not always fully describe the recruitment and training and other aspects of the programme development which might have an important effect on the outcome. Further findings from peer education in school settings showed that a substantial minority of students did not enjoy the peer-led interventions or learn anything new from them (Forrest *et al.*, 2002).

Why peer education approaches are useful

Understanding more about the practical considerations of developing and implementing peer education programmes helps in establishing successful projects. Harden *et al.* (1999) identified 15 high quality process evaluations, half addressing sexual health. Although these studies focused on different aspects of peer education programmes, limiting possibilities to draw conclusions for all types of peer approaches, the authors found a number of common issues outlined below.

Young people relate to peers as educators

Satisfaction and acceptability is associated with: being able to relate well to peer educators; perceiving them as credible sources of information; feeling relaxed during lessons; describing them as fun; appreciating not being lectured at and looked down on; feeling confident that peer educators would not breach any confidences (unlike teachers); feeling that peer educators did not act as 'if they knew it all' and that they understood young people's problems better than teachers.

However, some studies (Fox *et al.*, 1993; Schonbach, 1995; Strouse *et al.*, 1990) have shown that some young people were unhappy with aspects of peer education programmes. Some young men have expressed reservations about the way that peer educators deal with some emotive issues, like abortion, and the emphasis they placed on feelings and emotions. Other young people were uncomfortable when peer educators were shy or nervous. There were signs too that peer education may have a different appeal for young women and young men. In this case it has been suggested that boys enjoyed the relatively lax discipline imposed by peer educators but that this was at the expense of girls' sense of comfort and safety.

Young people find peer education methods acceptable and satisfactory

Peer educators, especially those working in formal settings like schools, often chose methods which some other sex educators feel less comfortable and confident about using, like role plays and small group activities and games. Young people often feel that these make for a better environment for talking about sex and relationships because it makes the information easier to digest and is potentially less intimidating than other more didactic teaching methods. Some research in schools suggests that some students see this choice of methods as a reflection of peer educators' understanding of how they like to learn, and recognition of how embarrassing sex and relationships can be (Forrest *et al.*, 2002).

Involvement in programmes enhanced the personal development of the peer educators

Many evaluations show that young people who become peer educators increase their knowledge, confidence and interpersonal skills as a result (for example, Phelps *et al.*, 1994; Strange *et al.*, 2002b). Peer education has been shown to increase their sense of maturity and sexual knowledge, enable peer educators to clarify their attitudes and values, and also boosts their confidence about managing their own relationships, as well as making them feel more confident about making presentations, giving information, and more empathetic towards teachers and other people who educate. There are also ongoing attempts to develop recognized qualifications, but this leads to tensions between establishing unnecessary formalities and therefore acting as a deterrent to some young people, and arriving at a transparent and meaningful system of accreditation, particularly in informal settings. It is inevitable that attempts to accredit peer educators will take us back to discussions about what exactly it is and how it functions. Without agreement on these matters agreement on assessment and accreditation is unlikely.

Peer education has the potential to reach groups of young people traditionally regarded as particularly at-risk and vulnerable to poor sexual health outcomes

In fact, it may be a particularly appropriate means according to the theoretical and historical background that places such a degree of emphasis on the empowerment of communities. However, it is very likely that these groups are better reached through outreach and community-based approaches rather than through formal settings. Experience of agencies like the Black Health Agency in the UK also suggest that particular attention needs to be given to building relationships within communities and there should be an acknowledgement of issues which have a high priority for the potentially peer educated. In this case, issues include experiences of racism and the development of a positive sense of identity.

It is particularly relevant when working with hard-to-reach groups to reflect on how peer educators, through their involvement with projects and programmes, negotiate the tensions between becoming an expert, and therefore potentially an outsider to their peer group, and remaining part of it. There are some hints in existing research that the perceived status of peer educators is associated with perceptions of their personal characteristics, motivations and the degree of trust the peer educated feel able to invest in them, but this remains to be explored more systematically.

Potential challenges for peer education

There may be limits to how far peer education conducted face-to-face can diffuse information among young people

Some research suggests that peer educators may not find it very easy to access other young people outside those that they set out to intervene with, their friends and other peer educators (Frankham, 1998). It is important to consider if other media, especially IT, offer opportunities for young people to make contact with peer educators.

Societal attitudes to sexuality impact on peer education as much as other approaches

There may be a reluctance to address potentially sensitive and complex issues that are found in this area. This reluctance is understandable in the current societal environment where there is little encouragement to discuss issues relating to sexuality openly. This is potentially compounded by certain settings, for example, schools, and certainly research by the school inspectorate in England suggests that other providers of sex education steer clear of these areas (OFSTED, 2002).

Tensions can exist between the methods and 'philosophy' of peer education approaches and traditional pedagogy in school-based programmes.

Teachers sometimes undermine peer educators' control over the content and organization of the lessons they provide, and some peer educators are seen as teachers by the young people they work with. Programmes can try to avoid this tension by setting out very clearly what role and responsibilities each has.

Conflicts can exist within projects between coordinators and their managers, and between young people and coordinators over their partnership

Conflicts tend to involve struggles about how resources were used and in which direction projects developed. While there does seem to be broad agreement that it is highly appropriate in peer education projects for peer educators to have some involvement in the direction of the work, the precise form that this takes is subject to variation at a local level. When projects are funded from statutory monies it is normal for the aims, objectives and ultimate responsibility and accountability to lie with a professional rather than with young people. It is also the case that the agenda in these situations is likely to be closely defined by the funder and that this will determine the focus on the project. This is clearly evident in the shift in emphasis from HIV/AIDS to teenage pregnancy between the 1980s and 1990s.

Recruitment can be a sensitive issue

Some young people may be more used to getting involved in projects and activities than others, and it can be seen as easier for young women to be seen to show an interest in sexual health than young men. The focus of the project, the kind of work it will involve and who is already involved will all have a bearing on whether young people will see it as relevant and interesting for them to be involved in or not. Similarity between peer educators and themselves might be less important to young people than the fact that they are confident and outgoing people (Strange *et al.*, 2002a). The timing of recruitment will also impact on recruitment (Strange *et al.*, 2002a), for example examinations or assessments will affect uptake.

Although most projects seem to negotiate any issues that arise from attracting too much interest from potential peer educators, there might be a need to screen and select from a pool of applicants, which presents project coordinators with the difficulties inherent in rejecting young people. Even where a formal screening and selection process is not instigated, field data from the RIPPLE trial suggests that some teachers in schools may actively encourage some young people and discourage others from volunteering as peer educators, according to whether they perceive them to be appropriate role models, reliable or overstretched by existing commitments.

Peer education may not be as cheap as first appears

Experience suggests that while peer education projects and programmes may be relatively cheap to establish they often imply hidden costs: the time of health promotion specialists, teachers and youth workers who coordinate projects in particular. In addition, while peer educators are positive about initial training, as they gather experience they may need support with issues like classroom management (in the context of schools) and handling questions from young people that arise outside the formal peer education programme.

Effectiveness may be affected by the organization of the intervention

However, there is still inadequate information to enable identification of benefits or disadvantages associated with particular organizational features of peer education interventions, although this does suggest that these are highly bound by the context. For example, it could be asked if there is an optimal size for intervention groups, ratio of peer educators to educated, or duration for interventions, or if the age gap between educators and educated makes a difference. The current reality seems to be that peer education projects and programmes operate within logistical and circumstantial constraints within which reference to these factors is implicit rather than explicit. One unfortunate effect of this may be that these constraints place severe limitations on the effectiveness of peer education, as has been suggested in the case of teacher-led sex education in schools (Wight *et al.*, 2002).

Conclusion

Despite the level of interest in peer education as a means of teaching sex education and sexual health promotion to young people, the approach is deeply affected by the general problems that afflict sexual health work. For example, political and moral sensitivities about who should teach young people about sex and when and what they should learn remain raw (Epstein and Johnson, 1998). In addition, the training of teachers and other relevant professionals in this area remains patchy and inconsistent (Forrest *et al.*, 2001), with the whole issue marginal in curricula in formal and informal educational settings (Regis *et al.*, 2000). And finally, sex education is prone to tapping into existing anxieties and difficulties associated with sexuality and gender experienced by young people (Measor *et al.*, 1996).

The answer to the fundamental question of whether peer education is an effective approach to sexual health promotion with young people has to remain, at best, a qualified yes. There is strong evidence that the processes involved are satisfactory and positive, especially for professionals and peer educators. The latter certainly seem to benefit in terms of self development and enhanced confidence although gains in terms of their own knowledge and changes in their behavioural intention seem less marked (Strange *et al.*, 2002a; Phelps *et al.*, 1994; Newitt *et al.*, 2000). There is also potential for formal qualifications or at least peer education contributing to school and college coursework.

However, the benefits for the peer educated in terms of learning and impact on behaviour should be drawn cautiously (Forrest *et al.*, 2002). Furthermore there are still weaknesses in theories and models of peer education, which are associated with the difficulties that arise from accounting for contextual influences. Our current understanding is limited and does not account for the complexities of intervention within the context of young peoples' lives. However, this is also the case for approaches including teacher-led sex education in schools (Wight *et al.*, 2002).

It might be that peer education in the UK has reached an important crossroads. The results of the RIPPLE study will influence assessments of what constitutes an effective programme. The expansion of existing projects and development of new ones may lead either to greater diversity of approach, or more similarity as tried and tested models become more attractive to funders. We may see struggles for ownership of the ethos of peer education. In terms of meeting the needs of young people we must hope for the development of more projects and programmes reflecting greater diversity in approach in order to maximize opportunities for them to access information, skills and support.

References

Abraham, C. and Sheeran, P. (1994) Modelling and modifying young heterosexuals' HIV-preventive behaviour; a review of theories, findings and educational implications. *Patient Education and Counselling* **23**: 173–86.

Backes, I. and Schonbach, K. with Buscher, I. *et al.* (2001) *Peer Education: A Manual for Practitioners*. Research and Practice of Sex Education and Family Planning, Federal Centre for Health Promotion, Cologne, Germany.

Backett-Milburn, K. and Wilson, S. (2000) Understanding peer education: insights from a process evaluation. *Health Education Research* **15**(1): 85–96.

Bandura, A. (1990) Perceived self-efficacy in the exercise of control over AIDS infection. *Evaluation and Program Planning* **13**: 9–17.

Campenhoudt, L., Cohen, M., Guizzardi, G. and Hausser, D. (1997) *Sexual Interactions and HIV Risk: New Conceptual Perspectives in European Research*. London: Taylor and Francis.

Charleston, S., Oakley, A., Johnson, A., Stephenson, J., Brodala, A., Fenton, K. and Petruckevitch, A. (1998) *Report on a Pilot Study for a Randomised Controlled Trial of Peer-Led Sex Education in Schools*. Social Science Research Unit, Institute of Education, London.

Clements, I. and Buczkiewicz, M. (1993) *Approaches to Peer-Led Health Education: A Guide for Youth Workers*. London: Health Education Authority.

Cowie, H. and Sharp, S. (1996) *Peer Counselling in Schools: A Time to Listen*. London: David Fulton.

Crosier, A., Goodrich, J., McVey, D., Forrest, S. and Dennison, C. (2002) *Involving Young People in Peer Education: A Guide to Establishing Sex and Relationships Peer Education Projects*. London: Department of Health.

DfEE (2000) *Sex and Relationship Education Guidance*. London: Department for Education and Employment.

Epstein, D. and Johnson, R. (1998) *Schooling Sexualities*. Buckingham: Open University Press.

Fishbein, M. (1990) AIDS and behaviour change: an analysis based on the theory of reasoned action. *Interamerican Journal of Psychology* **24**: 37–56.

Forrest, S., Strange, V. and Nash, T. (2001) Preparing teachers to provide effective sex and relationships education in secondary school. *Sex Education Matters* **27**: 3.

Forrest, S., Strange, V. and Oakley, A. (2002) A comparison of students' evaluations of a peer-delivered sex education programme and teacher-led provision. *Sex Education* **2**(3): 195–214.

Fox, J., Walker, B. and Kusher, S. (1993) *'It's Not a Bed of Roses'; Young Mother's Education Project Evaluation Report*. University of East Anglia, Norwich: Centre for Applied Research in Education.

Frankham, J. (1998) Peer education: the unauthorised version. *British Educational Research Journal* **24**(2): 179–93.

Harden, A., Weston, R. and Oakley, A. (1999) *A Review of the Effectiveness and Appropriateness of Peer-Delivered Health Promotion Interventions for Young People*. EPI-Centre, Social Science Research Unit, Institute of Education,

University of London.

Hartley-Brewer, E. (2002) *Stepping Forward: Working Together Through Peer Support*. London: National Children's Bureau.

Jaquet, S., Robertson, N. and Dear, C. (1996) *The Crunch*. Edinburgh: Fast Forward Positive Lifestyle.

Kleiber, D. and Pforr, P. (1995) Peer involvement: an approach to prevention and health promotion by young persons for young persons, in BZgA (ed.), *Learn to Love: Proceedings of the 1st European Conference on 'Sex Education for Adolescents'*, Cologne, Germany.

Measor, L., Tiffin, C. and Fry, K. (1996) Gender and sex education: a study of adolescent responses. *Gender and Education* 8(3): 275–88.

Mellanby, A. R., Phelps, F. A., Crichton, N. J. and Tripp, J. H. (1995) School sex education: an experimental programme with educational and medical benefit. *British Medical Journal* 311(7002): 414–17.

Mellanby, A. R., Rees, J. B. and Tripp, J. H. (2000) Peer-led and adult-led school health education: a critical review of available comparative research. *Health Education Research* 15(5): 533–45.

Newitt, K., Karp, M., McClure, A., Cowan, Y. and Ross, C. (2000) *Peer Education in the New Millennium: Guidelines For Practice*. Belfast: Eastern Health and Social Services Board.

OFSTED (2002) *Sex and Relationships*. London: OFSTED.

Phelps, F. A., Mellanby, A. R., Crichton, N. J. and Tripp, J. H. (1994) Sex education: the effects of a peer programme on pupils (aged 13–14 years) and their peer leaders. *Health Education Journal* 53: 127–39.

Prochaska, J. O. and DiClemente, C. (1986) Towards a comprehensive model of change, in W. R. Miller and N. Heather (eds), *Treating Addictive Behaviours: Processes of Change*. New York: Plenum.

Reeder, G. D., Pryor, J. B. and Harsh, L. (1997) Activity and similarity in safer sex workshops led by peer educators, *AIDS Education and Prevention*, Suppl. A: 77–89.

Regis, D., Lawrence, J. and Kanabus, A. (2000) A survey of sex education provision in secondary schools. Horsham: AVERT.

Rogers, E. M. (1983) *Diffusion of Innovations*. New York: Free Press.

Rosenstock, I. M. (1974) The health belief model and health preventive behaviour. *Health Education Monographs* 2: 354–86.

Rosenthal, D., Moore, A. and Flynn, I. (1991) Adolescent self-efficacy, self-esteem and sexual risk-taking. *Journal of Community and Applied Social Psychology*, 1: 77–88.

Schonbach, K. (1995) *Health Promotion and Peer Involvement for Youth*. Berlin: Themen and Konzepte.

Sciacca, J. P. (1987) Student peer health education: A powerful yet inexpensive helping strategy. *Peer Facilitator Quarterly* 5.

Social Exclusion Unit (1999) *Teenage Pregnancy*. London: The Stationery Office.

Strange, V., Forrest, S., Oakley, A. and the RIPPLE study Team (2002a) Peer-led sex education – characteristics of peer educators and their perceptions of the impact on them of participation in a peer education programme. *Health Education Research* 17(3): 327–37.

Strange, V., Forrest, S., Oakley, A. and the RIPPLE team (2002b) What influences peer-led sex education in the classroom? A view from the peer educators. *Health Education Research* 17(3): 339–49.

Strouse, J. S., Krajewski, L. A. and Gillin, S. M. (1990) Utilizing undergraduate students as peer discussion facilitators in human sexuality classes. *Journal of Sex Education and Therapy* 16(4): 227–35.

Svenson, G. (1998) *European Guidelines for Youth Aids Peer Education.* Sweden: University of Lund.

Taylor, S. E. (1986) *Health Psychology.* New York: Random Books.

Tones, B. K. and Tilford, S. (1994) *Health Education: Effectiveness, Efficiency and Equity.* London: Chapman and Hall.

Vygotsky, L. S. (1962) *Thought and Language.* Cambridge, Mass.: MIT Press.

Weare, K. (2000) *Promoting Mental, Emotional and Social Health: A Whole School Approach.* London: Routledge.

Wight, D., Abraham, C. and Scott, S. (1998) Towards a psycho-social theoretical framework for sexual health promotion. *Health Education Research* 13(3): 317–30.

Wight, D., Raab, G., Henderson, M., Abraham, C., Buston, K., Hart, G. and Scott, S. (2002) Limits of teacher delivered sex education: interim behavioural outcomes from a randomised trial. *British Medical Journal* 324, 15 June: 1430–5.

Guides and manuals supporting the development of peer education programmes and projects

Backes, I. and Schonbach, K. with Buscher, I. *et al.* (2001) *Peer Education: A Manual for Practitioners.* Research and Practice of Sex Education and Family Planning; Federal Centre for Health Promotion. Cologne, Germany.

Brodala, A. and Mulligan, J. (1999) *The Peer Aid Book: Approaches to Setting Up and Running Young People's Peer Education Projects.* London: CSV Education for Citizenship and the IBIS Trust.

Crosier, A., Goodrich, J., McVey, D., Forrest, S. and Dennison, C. (2002) *Involving Young People in Peer Education: A Guide to Establishing Sex and Relationships Peer Education Projects.* London: Department of Health.

Svenson, G. (1998) *European Guidelines for Youth Aids Peer Education.* Lund, Sweden: University of Lund. http://www.europeer.lu.se

14 'I Slept with 40 Boys in Three Months.' Teenage Sexuality in the Media: Too Much Too Young?

SUSAN BATCHELOR

with case study by

MARTIN RAYMOND

Key issues

- Attention to the diversity of form and focus within different media is crucial to understanding how teenage sexuality is represented.
- Young people are not passive dupes of media messages; they actively construct their own varied interpretations and understandings.
- Health educators need to be aware of both the richness and the limitations of current mainstream representation in order to work with and through the media.

Overview

This chapter will outline the main messages about sexuality and sexual health in media outlets consumed by young people, and offers some insight into how young people use and are affected by media sexual content. The extent to which the teen media deal with sex and related issues, such as contraception and STIs, will be explored before focusing on the potential influence of the media on how young people think about sexuality and how they behave sexually. Finally the implications for using the media to improve sexual health are explored.

Putting teen sex and the media in context

The mass media – television, magazines, newspapers, advertising, radio, music, films and the Internet – play an integral role in young people's lives. Young people aged from 6 to 17 living in the UK spend around five hours per day with one form of media or another (Livingstone and Bovill, 1999). What's more, evidence would suggest that this level of use is growing as forms of media proliferate (Livingstone, 2002). Young people today live in an increasingly complex, global media environment where new information and communication technologies – such as the Internet, digital television, interactive CD-ROMs and computer games – are becoming more personalized, more individualized and therefore less easy to regulate.

This diversification and multiplication of media forms means that while the mass media can play an important role in shaping young people's knowledge and attitudes toward sexuality (Brown *et al.*, 2002; Greenberg *et al.*, 1992), the messages they present can often be conflicting and confusing. In the UK in recent years we have seen vigorous debate concerning the perceived proliferation of images of teenage sex and sexuality in the mass media, particularly in magazines aimed at girls and young women. Much of this concern has centred on the belief that the media encourage young people to think that heterosexual intercourse before 16 is the norm and that young people may copy what they see (Millwood Hargrave and Halloran, 1996; Millwood Hargrave, 1999).

Given that young people themselves rank the media as a key source of sexual information (Todd *et al.*, 1999), it is important that health professionals are aware of how, where and whether young people come into contact with sound, reliable information about sex.

Ways in which teen sexuality is presented in the media

Despite current levels of concern and media usage among young people, there has been little UK research into what the media actually provide in terms of sexual health information (Bragg and Buckingham, 2002). Focusing on two main forms of teen media – teen television dramas and teen magazines – this section will examine what evidence exists in the UK, and look at research from elsewhere to establish the diverse media images that teenagers are exposed to.

Much of the existing research in this area originates in North America, particularly the USA and, whilst providing a useful background against which an understanding of young people and the media can be developed, cannot be unproblematically projected onto the British context. That said, teenagers are perhaps the first truly globally orientated audience sector (Langham Brown *et al.*, 1999), and many American-produced media are imported to the UK, particularly teen soaps. Another caveat we should note in reading the research findings that follow is that media sexual content is not fixed but varies substantially across formats and across time. Research focused on single forms of media and/or 'snapshot' samples does not address ongoing story lines or shifts in coverage over time, nor the ways in which particular media images are contextualized in relation to other media.

Teen drama

In their study of a one-week sample of Scottish media, Batchelor and Kitzinger (1999) found that the predominant portrayal of teenage sexuality on television aimed at teens involved conversations about sex, that is, people talking about the 'opposite sex', flirting or dating, male bravado and/or teasing and sexual negotiation. In interactions between the sexes, the general picture was of boys/men as pursuers and girls/women as the pursued. Male characters initiated most sexual behaviour and conversation, whereas females were depicted as responsible for managing male wants and limiting their access (see Box 14.1). Girls were also portrayed as being more interested in emotions and boys in sex, and whereas female characters were able to talk to their friends about the decision to have sex, male conversations tended to centre on boasting about sexual prowess. Hence young male sexuality was portrayed as physical and self-centred, whilst teenage female sexuality revolved around issues of emotionality and relational context.

No references to the physical consequences of sexual intercourse were found within Batchelor and Kitzinger's television sample. Likewise, contraception and protection against sexually transmitted infections (STIs) were never discussed and the only reference to contraceptive use within the 88½ hours of television viewed consisted of a one-and-a-half second shot of an open condom packet lying on a bedside table. No disabled, gay or lesbian teenagers were represented in the sample.

This supports findings from research conducted in North America. In their content analysis of sexual messages in teenagers' favourite primetime

---

Box 14.1 Teenage sexuality on television

Excerpt from USA teen drama, 'Sweet Valley High'

Liz:	Todd, wait… I've been thinking a lot about this and I'm just not sure. It's a big step for us. It would change everything.
Todd:	Liz, I don't want you to do anything you don't want to do.
Liz:	It's not just me – it's us. Do you really think we're ready for this?
Todd:	Well, I don't know.
Liz:	Don't you think it would be better if we had no doubts at all?
Todd:	Maybe you're right. [They embrace]

Excerpt from British soap, 'Family Affairs'

Donna:	We've been seeing each other for a week now. We should be past the stage of groping each other.
Benji:	Yeah? Well, I'm game if you are!
Donna:	[Slaps Benji's hand off her knee] No! I don't mean that! I mean talking to each other – like proper couples do. Getting to know each other.

Source: Batchelor and Kitzinger, 1999

television programmes in the USA, Cope-Farrar and Kunkel (2002) found that only about one in nine of the programmes that included sexual content (11 per cent) mentioned possible risks or responsibilities. STIs other than HIV and AIDS were almost never discussed, and characters involved in sexual behaviour rarely experienced any negative consequences (for example, unintended pregnancy) as a result of their actions. In other words, while 'television programming and advertising in general provide young people with lots of information about how to be sexy ... they provide little information about how to be sexually responsible' (Hayes, 1987: 91).

Magazines

Content analyses of magazines for girls and young women present a some-what different picture. A review of the role of teenage magazines in the sexual health of young people carried out by Kaye Wellings for the Teenage Magazine Arbitration Panel (TMAP) found the quality of information provided commendable, particularly in features designed to help young people adopt routine safer sex behaviours. Wellings noted that, compared with other agencies (for example, schools, official health education organizations), teenage magazines had an unparalleled 'capacity to discuss sex frankly and openly, to raise issues relating to sexual desire and pleasure and to provide role models with whom *young women* can identify' (Wellings, 1996: 17, emphasis added). Furthermore, she argued:

> magazines are in a strong position to be able to empower women, enabling them to make effective choices and exercise control in their own lives. They can also provide a language with which sex can be discussed and offer guidance on a 'script' for use in sexual encounters.
>
> (ibid.)

This conclusion was reiterated by Batchelor *et al.,* who found that 'amongst the humour and titillation some products provided useful information about sexual health and related issues' (forthcoming). These authors noted, however, that the quality of advice offered in teen magazines varied according to the different publications (see Box 14.2). Agony and health pages in girls' and young women's magazines offered the most detailed sexual health data, but publications aimed at a male audience were far less detailed and explicit. What's more, in asserting young women's right to determine 'how far' they went, publications reinforced stereotypes about the 'natural' behaviour of young men and boys, and in doing so depicted contraception, safer sexual practices and 'consent' as women's responsibility. A further reservation expressed by the researchers related to a failure to represent teenage diversity, since the young people depicted were overwhelmingly white, able-bodied, heterosexual and slim.

Box 14.2 Teenage sexuality in magazines

Article on kissing from teen magazine Mizz, *24 Mar–6 Apr 1999*

When you are really comfortable with someone, you can get a bit more intimate and open your mouth a little bit. If you like the lad a lot and feel relaxed with him, you may want to go a little further and French kiss. French kissing is when you open your mouth and caress the other person's lips and tongue with yours. While you do this you may feel the inside of their mouth too. It may sound a bit gross now, but it can leave you all floaty and happy after you have done it! Remember, you should only do it if really want to, though.

Letter to problem page from lads mag frOnt, *Apr 1999*

Reader: I find the thought of putting my mouth anywhere near her nether regions disgusting and she asks me to try it every time we're together. What should I do to avoid this fate worse than death?

Agony aunt: Do you think your nuts and bolts are so irresistible that she is drawn to them against her will? Or does she swallow her gagging instincts and pleasure your pendulum out of lurve and a sense of duty perchance? If you find women's organs so frightening then perhaps you too should call the above number [for the Lesbian and Gay Switchboard]. Otherwise get on your knees and do what she says.

Problem page 'Sexplanation' from teen magazine J-17, *Apr 1999*

Sexual intercourse with a girl under the age of 16 is illegal in Britain. This means that any boy or man is at risk of being prosecuted if there is enough evidence to prove he had sex with a girl under 16 years old – whether the girl wanted to have sex with him or not. And there have also been cases where older women have been sent to prison for having sex with boys aged under 16.

You can go to a clinic or GP surgery for help on any aspect of your health, regardless of your age. If you want advice on any aspect of sex, staff have to make sure that you are not a victim of child abuse. To do this, the doctor or nurse may ask you some questions about your health and then specific questions to make sure you understand the various issues around sex. These may include questions on contraception, the risks and benefits of any treatment they might give you, and whether or not you are able to discuss sex or contraception with your parents. The doctor then needs to consider whether your physical or mental health might suffer if you don't get advice, help or contraception and finally, what would be in your best interests.

All patients have the same right to confidentiality, whatever their age.

Box 14.2 continued

This means that doctors have to keep your personal information private unless there are exceptional circumstances. Only if something really awful were about to happen – like you were dying – would your doctor have to let your parents or other people know confidential details about you and your health.

Source: Batchelor and Kitzinger, 1999

Content analyses of US magazines present a similar picture. Comparing teen publications with magazines aimed at an older female audience, Walsh-Childers *et al.* (2002) found that teen titles were more likely to provide information on sexual health concerns. Among the sexual health topics discussed, pregnancy, contraception and HIV/AIDS were the most common, while abortion received very little attention. Perhaps unsurprisingly, the only sexual health topic that (adult) women's magazines were more likely to mention was planned pregnancy. The study also found evidence to suggest that the amount of space given to non-health sex topics versus sexual health articles had increased in both categories over the study period (1986–96).

To summarize, then, content analyses show that the media are full of sex – often presented in ways that glamorize the pleasurable aspects but rarely focus on the consequences of sexual relationships. Also, they suggest that sexual content is not uniformly depicted across media. This diversity makes the task of identifying media effects increasingly difficult.

Young people's interpretation of media content

One of the key issues in debates relating to sex in the media is to what extent the media influence teenagers' attitudes and behaviours. Research on young people's responses to media sexual content is sparse. This is partly due to the difficulties involved in documenting the effects of media on people's behaviour (Buckingham, 1993): in particular, difficulties in making causal links between viewing and behaviour (Zuckerman and Zuckerman, 1985). To do this effectively would require randomly assigning young people to watch specific programmes over long periods of time, while barring a comparable group from those shows – both improbable treatments given the pervasiveness of today's media sex content.

Consequently there is considerable debate concerning media effects, particularly their impact and influence upon young people. The media are now rarely conceptualized simply in terms of unidirectional impact on the audience. Emphasis is increasingly placed on how individuals construct their own meanings, in the diversity of reading and responses, and in how this then affects the communication process (Brown, 2000). Teenage audiences are particularly diverse, and young people pick and choose from a variety of images and messages. (A selection of young people's views are expressed in Box 14.3.)

One of the few studies of teenagers' reading of media content (carried out in the USA) found significant differences in interpretation of Madonna's music video, *Papa Don't Preach* (Brown and Schulze, 1990). Although most white girls thought the video depicted a young woman deciding to keep her unborn baby, black males said the woman was singing about wanting to keep her boyfriend, 'Baby'. Ward *et al.* (2002) also found discrepancies in the way in which US college students perceived sexual content in television sitcoms such as *Roseanne* and *Martin*. Compared with young men, young women in their study were more likely to think that the sexual scenes portrayed were realistic. The young men were less approving than the young women of relationship-maintaining behaviours (for example, jealous husband protecting wife) and were more approving of relationship threats (for example, man contemplating infidelity).

In her recent analysis of sexual self expression on teenage girls' internet home pages, Stern (1999) found girls critiquing the images they saw of themselves in the mass media and producing alternative versions of what sex and sexuality might be. This ability of young people to 'resist' media messages is a common line of defence used by magazine editors against criticisms that their publications encourage young people to think that heterosexual intercourse before 16 is the norm. Drawing on the concept of the active audience, they claim that their publications are full of humour and that teenage readers are more 'knowing' than social commentators give them credit for.

This is an argument taken up by McRobbie, who contends that 'the widespread use of irony and humour allows a space for distance and detachment from what is being normatively advocated, i.e. lots of sex' (McRobbie, 1996: 192). In other words, teenage consumers read media products tongue-in-cheek and are aware that the sexualized nature of the magazines is 'just a laugh'. Yet the degree to which readers are capable of reading reflexively is likely to be related to age and/or level of maturity, since irony may be lost on the average 16 year old. Regardless of the target audience, 'the fact is that magazines are read by younger readers than is stated and there may be evidence that they may take the views and behaviours of those magazines at face value' (Wellings, 1996:15).

Research carried out by the Glasgow Media Group has suggested that where people have no direct experience or other knowledge of an issue, the power of the media message is increased (Philo and McLaughlin, 1995). Conversely, people who have direct experience of an issue that conflicts with a media account are more likely to reject the media message (Philo, 1990). (An important exception to this is where media coverage raises great anxiety or fear, thereby overwhelming personal experience. See Philo, 1996.) This finding is supported by Brown *et al.* (1992), who found that girls with more actual sexual experience were more critical of media

---

Box 14.3 What young people say about media sexual content

I read *Bliss* for a laugh. I don't take it very seriously ... I do think that younger girls look to the problem pages for information and advice.... If there are girls that are easily influenced the magazine has quite a strong message about not having underage sex.

14 year old girl (quoted in Woods, 1997)

I think you feel uncool after reading such a magazine, but, there again, boys read all the girls' magazines ... it's our favourite reading on the bus in the morning. We just sit down and read all the problem pages. It's really amusing.... I think it's probably boys that need it more than girls to be honest, especially the boys I know.

16 year old boy (quoted in Forrest, 1997)

You see all these love scenes on TV and they are all panting away and saying that's lovely. And you think 'Oh!' But when it comes to the real thing it's a big disappointment. I think it's the mass media I get all my expectations from.

Young woman (quoted in Kent and Davis, 1992)

It's easy to point fingers at the media, I think. But there's also personal responsibility. Why should we blame magazines and TV and movies and books when they are a fine source of information? They're not lying about anything, but they're not giving us exactly what we want to hear. Well, that's why we need our parents, or that's when we need educators, teachers ... things like that to help us.

Young woman (quoted in Triese and Gotthoffer, 2002)

---

portrayals of sexuality, and Ward *et al.* (2002), who found that viewers who attribute a high degree of realism to television portrayals may be especially open to accepting accompanying messages.

Conclusion

What are the implications of these findings for sexual health professionals? Ways of working with the media are covered in the next section. Here, it is enough to say that policy makers and practitioners need to move beyond a purely defensive approach and beware of sweeping generalizations about 'harmful media effects'. As we have seen, recent studies suggest that the range of media available to young people today have become increasingly specialized (Brown, 2000), offering different audiences different kinds of content from which they pick and choose a variety of images and messages (Brown *et al.*, 1992). This points us to the importance of social context in understanding the influence of media content (Livingstone, 2002). Young people do not engage with the media in a vacuum, but rather the messages presented are mediated by personal experience and in interaction with significant others.

Working in the Field: A Practitioner's View

Case study by MARTIN RAYMOND

Working with and through the media

There are various ways of working with and through the media to promote sexual health, ranging from influencing the media (for example, regarding censorship), to using the media for direct messages (for example, advertising). It is accepted that there are limitations but also opportunities worth exploring. However, there are debates that are often played out through the media itself around censorship of sexual presentations in the media. Beyond clearly defined limits of what is acceptable in society and what material different age groups can access, there is little consensus about what is suitable fare for our teenagers. Indeed there is a growing debate about what is considered obscene. The British Board for Film Classification is constantly revising its position on what is considered acceptable and stimulates public debate on what limits society wishes to place on visual material. Remember that censorship also comes with the risk of making the racier parts of the media more attractive by being illicit.

Establishing guidelines for the media is just as difficult as constructing the more rigid absolutes of censorship. What can be relied upon is that the media will defend to the last its right to define its own ground rules rather than have them imposed by government. But given the freedom available on the wide-open spaces of the Internet, perhaps attempts to restrict access are the wrong approach.

What may be more effective is to equip young people with the skills to make sense of the media. By harnessing their natural fascination for virtually all media, we might be better served by giving them the ability to discriminate and deconstruct. Giving teenagers the knowledge to make the most of the sex education material that exists in the media and to be able to spot stereotyping and simplification elsewhere is better than an endless search for ways of thwarting knowledge.

As Felix Dennis, publisher of *Maxim* – a key 'lad mag' title – says: 'Our readers know us against the rest of the world' (BBC broadcast). We should learn something from the understanding that Dennis and others in the commercial world have for the needs of young men. In fact we can do much better. Rather than reinforcing unhelpful stereotypes that leave young people even more confined, we can give them an insight into the reality of relationships. We can give young people the ability to make sense of the media environment and help to make positive decisions about relationships. Most of all, they need to know it's not just *Maxim* on their side.

Finally actually using the media to promote messages and debate around sexual health has to be considered. Press and public relations work can have impact at both national and local level. Using the media to raise the awareness of sexual health matters can be effective but comes with risks since it is impossible to control the headlines. But by building positive relations, providing informative briefings and choosing media outlets carefully, you can begin to maximize the positives and minimize the negatives.

Using television advertising for sexual health promotion

So how can we use advertising to promote influence and change health related behaviour? At this point the apparent powerful effects of the media begin to evaporate. Suddenly we begin to talk in terms of limitations and restricted ambitions. However, provided that we are clear about the nature of our task there is every reason for health promoting organizations to take a walk on the wild side and develop their own media presence, as we have done in the Health Education Board for Scotland[1](HEBS) through the *Think about it* campaign described below.

A vital starting point is clarity of objective. The media can offer many things to health promotion, but one thing it can't provide is a magic solution to the ills of modern society. However, there are limited but important things that the media can do.

The media is useful in the transmission of information, which is often overlooked as an important function. Surveys regularly confirm that levels of knowledge on sexual health matters are very high among young people (Todd *et al.*, 1999). But while information is not all there is to responsible sexual behaviour, it is a vital precondition. So the media can be used for example, to draw young people's attention to changing patterns of STIs and the relevance to them.

Media initiatives also have a history of influencing attitudes but this takes mass media tools to the very limits of their effectiveness. Certainly the one thing that the media is not very good at is changing behaviour. Commercial marketing operates on the principle that media communications is one part of a combined effort involving that product itself, the places you can buy it and the activities of competitors. Isolating the effects of advertising is a sophisticated but ultimately inexact science.

Advertising makes its potentially biggest but most subtle contribution to health promotion in the area of popular culture. As the media fragments through channel multiplication, advertising, football and soaps are the few shared media experiences that are left. Advertising can both shape and reflect modern culture as surely as any other feature of society. So health needs to be there, part of that shared media mix, because being there is almost as important as the content of the advertising itself.

The media can also be used to ask penetrating questions about sex and relationships, which are in fact especially relevant to balance the ubiquitous presence of sex to sell products in virtually every market sector. Indeed this is the main aim of the *Think about it* campaign which literally asks young people to think about the impact of various health related behaviours on a range of physical, emotional and social outcomes.

Young people and the media

Despite the fact that commercial advertising has much greater budgets, good social marketing messages have often enjoyed a much higher margin of awareness because the audience recognizes that it is appreciably about something more important than commerce. The topic matter of health is universally interesting, even if it is not universally relevant. Teenagers are especially interested in the media and traditionally recall advertising at a much higher level of detail.

This is in part because for teenagers the world of the media has a unique excitement and resonance. The media is their world in a way that adult dominated environments like the home and school are not. They are aware of the huge energy and financial investment that goes into parting them from their own or their parents' money. All that – just for them! There is no more appreciative audience for advertising, and none so fiercely critical. So it is vital that the content of sexual health advertising is relevant and worthwhile in the eyes of the consumer.

Case study: *Think about it*

Think about it is an integrated teen health media initiative, which covers issues like drugs, alcohol and smoking as well as sexual health. But all advertisements are linked by common themes, the strongest being the role of relationships in determining how teenagers make/don't make decisions about their health. The adverts all challenge young people to think about the consequences of a particular health-related behaviour in relation to emotional, social or physical outcomes with the end line consistently being *Think about it*.

The development of a strand of sexual health advertising within the *Think about it* format began with extensive research among the target audience of 14 to 16 year olds. Before any script was written the key issues for teenagers were teased out. Groups spoke of the confusion of making sense of relationships, sexual drives and of coping with the expectations of peer groups (Wade, 1996; Reid, 2001).

Our research also uncovered respectable levels of knowledge but a yawning void of understanding of what was the best way to handle relationships. 'What do I say next?' 'What do I *do* next?': apparently simple but actually uniquely profound questions. Advertising cannot offer answers to these questions, but it can help ask more helpful questions and offer a range of options. It also has the potential to frame the questions in a new way. Young people in our groups kept returning to the emotional promise and risks of relationships. Picking up an infection is serious but not perhaps as serious as damaged self-esteem: certainly not from the perspective of teenagers themselves, whose priorities do not necessarily reflect a public health agenda.

The other gap that rapidly became apparent was the huge gulf separating the genders at this age. Attempting to understand the language of the other gender and translating stereotyped expectations into the real world, exercises the minds of teenagers more than any other factor.

The eventual advertisement produced by HEBS, developed as a two-part exploration of a single episode, explored all of these key issues (see Box 14.4). It immediately achieved high levels of awareness, and qualitative responses from teenagers focused on its realism and complexity.

What have we learnt?

It is first and foremost vital to ensure the inclusion of relevant issues for the target audience. Research with the audience is one of the most effective ways of hearing their voice and reflecting the key issues from the perspective of young people. However, ensuring the inclusion of relevant issues is not in itself enough to engage the interest of teenagers. The tone of voice employed is just as significant as the content, if not more so. The audience can accept a bit of authority, but there are so many apparent sources of advice and information on sex in the playground and in cyberspace, teenagers need to know whom they can trust. Often this will be based on a long-standing relationship between the 'brand' and the audience. But that authority cannot tip over into authoritarianism. Being told what to do is not compatible with being an adolescent: for example, the underpinning principle of *Think about it* is to encourage teenagers to see where their own responsibilities begin and end.

But that doesn't mean aping teenagers or attempting to be too cosy. The tone can be challenging and questioning. It can acknowledge the uncertainty of adolescence without becoming too conspiratorial. The credibility of the messenger is also vital: young people need to see the source organization as in tune with their needs and attitudes. Regular tracking of HEBS advertising showed that young people saw the organization as innovative, authoritative and 'on our side', all of which helps in getting the message across. Achieving this kind of brand identity takes time and may be challenging, especially for organizations linked to government or to institutions, which may be regarded as trying to control or preach to young people, but it is an essential foundation to effective work in this area.

Box 14.4 HEBS teenage sexual health and relationships advertisements
His Story and *Her Story* scripts

This commercial is filmed entirely from the narrator's point of view. We
see the world through **his** eyes

Vision	Audio
We open on a blue screen and title appears: HIS STORY.	
We are at a teenage party. We see a girl the other side of the room, she smiles at us.	BOY'S VOICE: I knew her a bit from school, I'd always fancied her.
We go over to her. She is pleased to see us, very chatty. (picture fades)	I got up the courage to go over, she was really friendly, I wasn't sure what to say.
Fade up to her on the dance floor, dancing very enthusiastically. (picture fades)	She was a real laugh, I felt a bit boring.
Fade up to her standing in a corner. She is drinking and chatting flirtatiously.	She seemed to really like me though.
We come closer until we are right up to her face. (picture fades)	We snogged, it was brilliant.
We look across the room. A group of boys are winking and making suggestive signs. (picture fades)	My mates were all egging me on.
We see her looking at him with affection. (picture fades)	She seemed really keen.
We are now going upstairs.	I didn't really want to do it but I didn't want her to think I was a wimp.
We open a door and go inside, the girl follows. Picture fades to black.	Somehow we just ended up upstairs.

Box 14.4 (continued)

This commercial is filmed entirely from the narrator's point of view. We see the world through **her** eyes.

Vision	*Audio*
Open on a blue screen and title appears: HER STORY.	
We are at a teenage party. We see a boy the other side of the room looking in our direction.	GIRL'S VOICE: I knew him a bit from school, a lot of the girls fancied him.
He comes towards us and says hello, he is quite shy.	I couldn't believe it when he came over.
We see the boy nodding. (picture fades)	I was really nervous and talked non-stop.
Now we are dancing with him. He is a bit awkward but tries to act cool and looks around quite a bit. (picture fades)	He was really cool on the dance floor, I went right over the top, trying to impress him.
Now we are in a dark corner, he is now flirting more obviously. We see another girl shoot an envious glance our way. (picture fades)	I knew my mates were dead jealous.
He comes right up close to us. picture fades)	Then we snogged, it was nice.
Now we are following him upstairs.	He said let's go upstairs, I wanted to say no but I didn't want him to think I was boring.
We follow him into a bedroom. (fade to black)	
Now we are pulling on clothes. We look towards the bed, the boy is lying there expressionless. We open the door and leave.	Afterwards he didn't speak to me at all. I was really upset. I've never felt so bad.
We fade to blue and line appears: THINK ABOUT IT. Followed by HEBS and website address.	

Notes

1 HEBS has since combined with the Public Health Institute Scotland to become NHS Health Scotland.

References

Batchelor, S. and Kitzinger, J. (1999) *Teenage Sexuality in the Media*. Edinburgh: Health Education Board for Scotland.

Batchelor, S., Kitzinger, J. and Burtney, E. (forthcoming) *Representing Young People's Sexuality in the 'Youth' Media'*. Health Education Research.

Bragg, S. and Buckingham, D. (2002) *Young People and Sexual Content on Television: A Review of the Research*. London: Broadcasting Standards Commission.

Brown, J. D. (2000) Adolescents' sexual media diets. *Journal of Adolescent Health*, **27**S: 35–40.

Brown, J. D., Barton White, A. and Nikopoulou, L. (1992) Disinterest, intrigue, resistance: early adolescent girls' use of sexual media content, in B. S. Greenberg, J. D. Brown and N. Buerkel-Rothfuss (eds), *Media, Sex and the Adolescent*. New Jersey: Hampton Press.

Brown, J. D. and Keller, S. N. (2000) Can the mass media be healthy sex educators? *Family Planning Perspectives* **32**(5): 255–6.

Brown, J. D. and Schultze, L. (1990) The effects of race, gender and fandom on audience interpretation of Madonna's music videos. *Journal of Communication* **40**: 88–102.

Brown, J. D., Steele, J. R., Walsh-Childers, K. (eds) (2002) *Sexual Teens, Sexual Media: Investigating the Media's Influence on Adolescent Sexuality*. Mahwah, NJ: Lawrence Erlbaum.

Buckingham, D. (ed.) (1993) *Reading Audiences: Young People and the Media*. Manchester: Manchester University Press.

Cope-Farrar, K. and Kunkel, D. (2002) Sexual messages in teens' favorite prime-time television programs, in J. D. Brown, J. R. Steele and K. Walsh-Childers (eds), *Sexual Teens, Sexual Media: Investigating the Media's Influence on Adolescent Sexuality*. Mahwah, NJ: Lawrence Erlbaum.

Forrest, S. (1997) Confessions of a middle shelf magazine shopper. *Journal of Contemporary Health* **5**: 10–13.

Greenberg, B. S., Brown, J. D. and Buerkel-Rothfuss, N. (eds) *Media, Sex and the Adolescent*. New Jersey: Hampton Press.

Haffner, D. W. (ed.) (1995) *Facing Facts: Sexual Health for America's Adolescents*. New York: SIECUS.

Hayes, C. D. (ed.) (1987) *Risking the Future: Adolescent Sexuality, Pregnancy and Childbearing*. Washington, DC: National Academy Press.

Kent, V. and Davis, M. (1992) *Social Interaction Routines in Heterosexual Encounters of Young People. Talking About It*. London: Health Education Authority.

Livingstone, S. (2002) *Young People and New Media*. London: Sage.

Livingstone, S. and Bovill, M. (1999) *Young People New Media*. London School of Economics and Political Science.

McKay, J. (1998) Dear Tony, can reading stuff like this make me pregnant? *The Scotsman*, 19 Nov.

McKay, J. (1999) *Manuals for Courtesans.* Paper presented at AJE conference 7 May 1999.

McRobbie, A. (1996) More!: new sexualities in girls' and women's magazines, in J. Curran, D. Morley and V. Walkerdine (eds), *Cultural Studies and Communications.* London: Hodder Arnold.

Millwood Hargrave, A. (1999) *Sex and Sensibility.* London: Broadcasting Standards Commission.

Millwood Hargrave, A. and Halloran, J. (1996) *Young People and the Media.* London: Broadcasting Standards Commission.

Philo, G. (1990) *Seeing and Believing: the Influence of Television.* London: Routledge.

Philo, G. (ed.) (1996) *Media and Mental Distress.* Harlow: Longman.

Philo, G. and McLaughlin, G. (1995) The British media and the Gulf War, in G. Philo (ed.), *Glasgow Media Group Reader Vol. 2: Industry, Economy, War and Politics.* London: Routledge.

Ralph, S. Langham Brown, J. and Lees, T. (eds) (1999) *Youth and The Global Media: Papers from the 29th University of Manchester Broadcasting Symposium.* Luton: University of Luton Press.

Reid, M. (2001) *HEBS Post Test Research Debrief.* Glasgow: Margaret Reid Research.

Stern, S. (1999) Adolescent girls' expression on WWW home pages: a qualitative analysis. *Convergence* 5(4): 22-41.

Teenage Magazine Arbitration Panel (1996) *Guidelines for Coverage of Sexual Subject Matter in Teenage Magazines.* London: TMAP.

Todd, J., Currie, C. and Smith, R. (1999) *Health Behaviours of Scottish School-children, Technical Report 2: Sexual Health in the 1990s.* University of Edinburgh: Research Unit in Health and Behavioural Change.

Triese, D. and Gotthoffer, A. (2002) Stuff you couldn't ask your parents: teens talking about using magazines for sex information, in J. D. Brown, J. R. Steele and K. Walsh-Childers (eds), *Sexual Teens, Sexual Media: Investigating the Media's Influence on Adolescent Sexuality.* Mahwah, NJ: Lawrence Erlbaum.

Wade, C. (1996) *Concept Development Teenage Health Campaign.* Fife: Clare Wade Research.

Walsh-Childers, K., Gotthoffer, A. and Lepre, C. R. (2002) From 'just the facts' to 'downright salacious': teens' and women's magazine coverage of sexual health, in J. D. Brown, J. R. Steele and K. Walsh-Childers (eds), *Sexual Teens, Sexual Media: Investigating the Media's Influence on Adolescent Sexuality.* Mahwah, NJ: Lawrence Erlbaum.

Ward, L. M., Gorvine, B. and Cytron-Walker, A. (2002) Would that really happen? Adolescents' perceptions of sexual relationships according to prime-time television, in J. D. Brown, J. R. Steele and K. Walsh-Childers (eds), *Sexual Teens, Sexual Media: Investigating the Media's Influence on Adolescent Sexuality.* Mahwah, NJ: Lawrence Erlbaum.

Wellings, K. (1996) *The Role of Teenage Magazines in the Sexual Health of Young People.* London: TMAP.

Woods, J. (1997) Sassy and sexy, but are today's 'girl power' magazines problem pages? *The Scotsman*, 24 Apr.

Wray, J. and Steele, J. (2002) Girls in print: figuring out what it means to be a girl, in J. D. Brown, J. R. Steele and K. Walsh-Childers (eds), *Sexual Teens,*

Sexual Media: Investigating the Media's Influence on Adolescent Sexuality. Mahwah NJ: Lawrence Erlbaum.

Zuckerman, D. M. and Zuckerman, B. S. (1985) Television's impact on children. *Pediatrics* 75: 233–40.

Further reading and websites

Further reading

For a recent edited collection exploring the sexual content of USA mass media and its influence in the lives of adolescents, see: Brown, J. D., Steele, J. R. and Walsh-Childers, K. (eds) (2002) *Sexual Teens, Sexual Media: Investigating the Media's Influence on Adolescent Sexuality.* Mahwah, NJ: Lawrence Erlbaum.

A useful review of the research on media effects can be found in: Livingstone, S. (1996) On the continuing problem of media effects, in J. Curran and M. Gurevitch (eds), *Mass Media and Society.* London: Arnold.

Websites

Children's Express UK
http://childrens-express.org
Children's news agency that empowers children as journalists. Includes a range of stories relating to sexual health researched and written by children.

Centre for the Study of Children, Youth and Media
http://www.ccsonline.org.uk/mediacentre/
Research centre based at the Institute of Education, University of London. Includes details of research projects, including ongoing study into 'Young People's Responses to Sexual Content on Television'.

Lovelife
http://www.playingsafely.co.uk
Sexual health site produced by Health Promotion England and aimed at young adults (16–24 years).

Media Education UK
http://www.mediaed.org.uk
Media literacy site with materials for teaching and learning about media production and analysis.

UK Children and Media Network
http://www.jiscmail.ac.uk/lists/CHILDREN-MEDIA-UK.html
On-line discussion forum for academics, regulators and those working in the media industries.

15 What Works and What Counts: The Role of Evidence and the Voice of Young People

MARY DUFFY and

ELIZABETH BURTNEY

Introduction

The contributions in this book demonstrate the complexity of young people's sexual health and the range of issues underlying a comprehensive and effective approach to supporting young people in making informed, healthy, safe and fulfilling choices about their sexual behaviour. They show that sexual health is affected by individual, familial, social, environmental and political influences, the relative weight of which may vary for different groups. The classic model developed for health in general illustrates these layers of influence (Figure 15.1).

This book also shows the importance of evidence when planning and implementing effective and efficient responses at both policy and practice level. In the UK the emphasis is increasingly on evidence-informed decision making, with the Modernizing Government agenda arguing that policy should build on the best available evidence about what works. The same drive to base action on supporting evidence is occurring at a practice level, in particular within the health sector. However, questions about what constitutes evidence remain, both within and across professional spheres.

The chapters draw on wide sources of evidence to present challenges and potential solutions with regard to promoting the sexual health of young people. Given the interaction between the layers of influence outlined above, they acknowledge that identifying the most effective approaches for influencing the choices that young people make or have available to them is difficult.

In all the chapters, the evidence discussed includes the views of young people themselves, gathered through surveys, consultation exercises and various forms of qualitative research. Taking account of these views is increasingly regarded as central to ethical and effective practice and policymaking, pushed forward in the UK by a range of statutory and voluntary sector initiatives. Indeed, there are even specific posts set up to advise national and local govern-

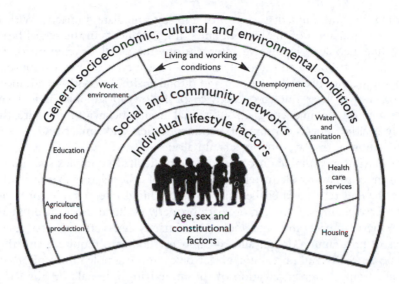

Figure 15.1 Factors influencing individual health

Source: Dahlgreen and Whitehead, 1991

ment on the best ways in which to engage with young people and families in order to formulate action plans sensitive to their needs and priorities (and therefore more likely to have the desired impact).

Rather than attempting to draw out all the lessons from the preceding sections, the rest of this chapter focuses on a more general discussion of issues relating to evidence and to user involvement. It builds on a paper by Duffy and McNeish (2003).

The importance of what works

What works is about outcomes

It is important to recognize that not everything that is done to improve sexual health outcomes for young people has the desired effect. Some interventions have more modest effects than intended; some have unintended (and often unmeasured) negative effects. Others may achieve positive outcomes but at a cost that could fund cheaper programmes achieving similar or better results. Some effective interventions to improve sexual health overall may even increase inequalities between groups, improving outcomes for some groups more than for others. In other words, social interventions to improve health, however well intentioned, can result in harm to individuals and wasteful resource allocation (Roberts, 2002).

In order to know whether something works, a clear specification of outcomes and a commitment to measuring these is required. This means moving beyond immediate outputs and intermediate impacts. Without critical examination of the bottom line – improvements in the sexual health of young people – ineffective interventions may well be continued. For example, distributing educational materials (outputs) is a common approach in many areas of health promotion and public health, but without additional approaches such as one-to-one advice or follow-up support, it is a very poor method for impacting on individual health behaviour. Despite this, many health agencies continue to produce leaflets and similar resources for distribution or display, often in a stand-alone way.

Specifying measurable outcomes can be difficult. In complex social interventions it is hard to adequately take account of other factors that may influence the end result and challenging to track things over a sufficient period to observe changes. Often, in order to properly evaluate short, medium and longer term impacts and outcomes and ultimately assess effectiveness, special types of programme design and research methods are required, and these can be expensive and unrealistic. Nevertheless, even simple interventions can benefit from clearer articulation of the underlying rationale or 'theory' of how change will happen and by sharper thinking about outcomes. This means being explicit about the steps by which a stated set of effects is to be achieved and measuring progress towards these.

What works isn't always what seems obvious

In earlier sections we discussed how evidence is never the main factor influencing the decisions that policy makers and practitioners make about issues relating to the sexual health of young people. However, taking account of a range of sources of evidence is likely to improve the chances of devising an effective project or programme. Searching for lessons from previous work, and in some instances from other countries, can help to challenge 'gut reactions' about what seems to be the obvious response.

For example, targeting health interventions in disadvantaged areas seems an obvious way of addressing inequalities and indeed has been the basis of some major initiatives. However, background analysis shows that many disadvantaged children do not live in 'poor' areas and therefore may be missed by these types of targeted programmes. Similarly, while condom distribution might seem like an obvious solution to curb rising STI rates, whether it actually has an effect depends on whether the condoms are used. This in turn depends on knowing the protective effects of condoms, knowing how to use them, having the confidence to carry them, and possessing the skills and confidence to negotiate their use in sexual situations.

What works isn't necessarily about 'health'

Sexual health can be improved through changes at many points in the system and often it is multifaceted, cross-sectoral action that brings the greatest benefits. For example, planning to avoid early parenthood is closely linked with having a stake in the future, a sense of hope and expectation of inclusion in society (UNICEF, 2001). This takes into account education, inequalities and social inclusion agendas, and requires action in schools, families and other arenas beyond the health service. And in terms of the overarching impact of poverty on sexual health and other outcomes, it is fiscal policy and changes to the welfare system that may offer most hope for reducing the differences between groups demonstrated throughout this book.

What could work isn't always what does work

While understanding whether something works is critical, it is also important to understand how it works, or why it doesn't work in some contexts. Sometimes the success of an intervention in one area may be due to aspects of the local community or the profile and approach of key workers. Without an appreciation of these process issues, interventions that could have a positive impact may not succeed. That is why a full description of all aspects of design and delivery of a given project or programme is an essential aspect of any comprehensive evaluation.

Similarly, infrastructure issues sometimes create a barrier to success for interventions that in principle could work. For example, intensive one-to-one support from health professionals during pregnancy and after delivery for women from deprived backgrounds may lead to better health outcomes for their children, but the ability to deliver such an intervention depends on having sufficient appropriately trained staff in place.

We don't always do what works

Decisions are often influenced by what is compelling (what 'tells a good story'); advocacy for certain approaches, brought to bear through consultation processes and through direct lobbying, can have a major impact. Issues of resource allocation also influence decisions, as does the perceived acceptability of proposed interventions to those receiving them. Such factors generally weigh much heavier in the decision-making process than an objective appraisal of research evidence (Davies *et al.*, 2000).

At a policy level in particular, politics inevitably play a part. In the UK in the 1980s, for example, the emphasis was less on tackling underlying structural factors leading to different health outcomes than on individual behaviour choices in relation to health. The rhetoric focused on individual responsibility (and therefore blame) for health outcomes and on 'health variations' rather than the now familiar health inequalities. The nature of political leadership at that time meant that certain types of responses were preferred, in some cases despite evidence of need and effectiveness.

In the sexual health field specifically, despite evidence that abstinence programmes are not more effective at improving sexual health outcomes for young people, in the USA vocal support from politically powerful groups and a number of legislative and funding decisions, all stemming from an underlying current of social and political conservatism, have allowed them to flourish. As Chapter 5 outlines: 'only 14 per cent of schools [in the USA] have "truly comprehensive" policies, despite evidence that the vast majority of teachers, parents and young people prefer more comprehensive coverage.'

We don't always know what works

Despite calls for action based on evidence of effectiveness, in many instances we simply do not know what works, or what is likely to work best in a given situation. In such cases, and in particular where there are obvious problems, inaction is not an option. The responsible course is to make best use of what evidence there is available, to address what we do know as a priority, and to take calculated risks in experimenting with new approaches.

Where innovative interventions are being tried, it is crucial that monitoring and evaluation systems are in place. These should help to record the process of implementation and assess the short, medium and longer term impacts and outcomes, generating evidence against which effectiveness can be judged and which can be used to inform subsequent interventions. Such a systematic approach to describing, implementing, monitoring and evaluating interventions has value at all levels of action – in terms of policy, programme development and project delivery. The teenage pregnancy strategy in England (Social Exclusion Unit, 1999) is a good example at a policy level of a longer term investment in improving sexual health, where innovative practice is encouraged, long-term goals set and an evaluation plan established. At a programme level, the Youth Development Centres being piloted across England from 2003 also seek to innovate in terms of improving sexual health outcomes, building on promising results from similar work in the USA and attaching independent evaluators to the development of the initiative from the outset.

Listening to the voices of young people

The United Nations Convention on the Rights of the Child (1989) states that young people have a right to express their views on matters affecting them and that these views should be given due weight. This drive to engage more meaningfully with young people and to take adequate account of their needs and preferences is reflected in many areas of international policy, although implementation lags significantly behind rhetoric.

Under the New Labour political agenda in the UK, there is an increasing recognition of the views of those at whom policy approaches and practice responses are aimed. As discussed above and in previous sections, this is evident in health and many other areas. For example, in UK Children's Fund work, where there is a target relating to teenage pregnancy, direct engagement with young people in developing appropriate responses is a fundamental requirement, and success in achieving this dialogue with young people, and in taking the findings of this dialogue into account in programme delivery, is measured through local and national level evaluation. As a result, there has been a proliferation of 'Voices' and similar initiatives set up to engage directly with young people, and to help create links between professional decision makers and those whom their decisions affect.

Also in the health field, the National Service Framework for children, young people and families sets out a requirement for meaningful consultation with service users. Although this focuses on hospital services, its aims reflect those now typical of many developments in that there is a commitment to offering:

- integrated and coordinated care around needs of children, young people and families
- engagement with children, young people and families as active partners in decisions about their health and care
- participation with children, young people and families in designing NHS and social care services that are accessible, respectful, empowering, follow best practice in obtaining consent and provide effective response to needs
- appropriate locations and environments that are safe and well suited to the age and stage of development.

In relation to sexual health specifically, a range of documents now present, often in their own words, the views of young people (for example, Mullins and McCluskey, 2000; Children in Scotland *et al.*, 2002) and consultation phases direct with young people are common in policy and practice development.

Consulting in a non-tokenistic way with end users, especially children, can be challenging. It requires new ways of working and can throw up difficulties for project planning and implementation. Moreover, meaningful consultation sometimes uncovers differences between the experiences and views of young people and those of parents and professionals, and this can lead to conflict and difficulties regarding how best to address issues.

However, done effectively consultation often shows a lot of consistency between young people's views and those of the professionals. The current holistic focus at a national policy level and the emphasis on understanding health and related issues in their broader context are well understood by many young people. For example, when asked about threats to their health and things that improve wellbeing, young people talk about cutting down on risky behaviours but also about having better relationships, more money and safer communities (Barnardo's, 2001).

The sophisticated way in which many young people understand what impacts on their sexual health should be no surprise given that they are the expert witnesses on their own lives and on how things could be different.

Bearing this in mind, and seeing young people's views as a source of evidence to be taken into account alongside other important sources, can make consultation processes seem less threatening.

Conclusion

Identifying what works is fraught with difficulties. Research data are often unavailable, uncertain or inapplicable and there are never enough resources to tackle every issue adequately. The challenge for those working on social interventions to reduce inequalities in young people's health is to make best use of the research evidence that is available, be explicit about the intended outcomes of their programmes and the logic behind these, and be more rigorous about measuring and reporting effects. Yet at the same time as 'hardening' on issues of impacts and outcomes, a broader approach is required to take account of the views of end users as a legitimate form of evidence, critical to obtaining a full picture of what is required to make a difference.

References

Barnardo's (2001) *Whose Government is it Anyway?* Ilford: Barnardo's.

Children in Scotland, FPA (2002) *Sexpression.* Edinburgh: Children in Scotland.

Dahlgreen, G. and Whitehead, M. (1991) *Policies and Strategies to Promote Social Equality in Health.* Stockholm: Institute for Further Studies.

Davies, H. T. O., Nutley, S. and Smith, P. C. (2000) *What Works? Evidence-Based Policy and Practice in Public Services.* Bristol: Policy Press.

Duffy, M. and McNeish, D. (2003) Child health: what works and what counts. *Issues in Health Sector Reform*: 95–98.

Mullins, A. and McCluskey, J. (2000) *Teenage Mothers Speak for Themselves.* London: NCH Action for Children.

Roberts, H. (2002) Reducing inequalities in child health, in D. McNeish, T. Newman, H. Roberts (eds), *What Works for Children.* Milton Keynes: Open University Press/Barnardo's.

Social Exclusion Unit (1999) *Teenage Pregnancy.* London: The Stationery Office.

UNICEF (2001) A league table of teenage births in rich nations, *Innocenti Report Card No. 3.* Florence, Italy: UNICEF Innocenti Research Centre.

Name Index

All authors of papers and books cited are listed here, with co-authors referenced regardless of whether their name is cited when the work is mentioned in the text, but authors of edited collections from which specific articles are cited are not referenced. Titles of works are listed only when an author is not listed. Titles of organizations are listed here; specific laws are listed in the subject index.

A

A PAUSE 183–4
Aapola, S. 11, 12
Abma, J. C. 82, 94
Abortion Supervisory Committee (ASC) (New Zealand) 87–8, 92
Abraham, C. 16, 17, 18, 22, 25, 26, 27, 29, 119, 127, 141, 146, 153, 181, 187, 189, 205, 213, 214, 216
Acheson, D. 95, 97
Adler, N. E. 21, 28
Advocates for Youth 84, 92
Aggleton, P. 65, 75, 119, 121, 127, 195, 199
Alagiri, P. 93, 181, 188
Alan Guttmacher Institute (AGI) 83, 84, 93
All-Party Parliamentary Group on AIDS (APPGA) 158, 166
Allen, I. 65, 76
Amos, A. 8, 13
ANCHARD 89, 90, 93
Anderson, C. W. 35, 37
Ann Craft Trust 153
Annual Surveillance Report (Australia) 89, 93
Antal, A. 36, 37
APPGA see All-Party Parliamentary Group on AIDS
ASC see Abortion Supervisory Committee
Australian Bureau of Statistics 89, 93
Australian Federation of AIDS Organizations 90

Australian National Council for HIV, Hepatitis C and Related Diseases see ANCHARD

B

Bacchi, C. 6, 12
Backes, I. 205, 216
Backett–Milburn, K. 214
Bailey, J. 115, 121–2, 123, 125–6
Bandura, A. 191, 199, 214
Barnardo's 239, 240
Barton White, A. 223, 231
Batchelor, S. xi, 24, 27, 39, 57, 117, 118, 126, 170, 171, 218, 221–2, 231–2
Bauman, K. E. 193, 200
Bearinger, L. H. 193, 200
Bearman, P. 84, 93, 193, 200
Beets, G. 65, 68, 76
Beuhring, T. 193, 200
Beyond Barriers 124
Biddulph, M. 122, 125, 156, 158, 166
Biehal, N. 95, 97, 102, 112
BILD 153
Birmingham Specialist NHS Community Trust 137
Bisazza, P. 146, 150
Black Health Agency 137–8
Blair, Tony 57
Blake, S. xi, 137, 156, 157, 158, 161, 166
Bloxham, S. 65, 76
Blum, R. W. 193, 200
Bob and Rose 118
Bok, I. A. 193, 200
Bovill, M. 217, 231
Bowe, K. 96, 98
Bradby, H. 23, 27
Bragg, S. 218, 231
Brannen, J. 22, 25, 27
Bremberg, S. 95, 98
British Board for Film Classification 225
British Council 140, 150
Broad, B. 103, 113

241

Subject index